MY BREASTS, MY CHOICE
Journeys Through Surgery

MY BREASTS,
My Choice

JOURNEYS
THROUGH
SURGERY

*Barbara Brown,
Maureen Aslin &
Betsy Carey*

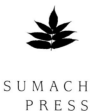

SUMACH
PRESS

2003 NATIONAL LIBRARY OF CANADA CATALOGUING IN PUBLICATION

My breasts, my choice: journeys through surgery / edited by Barbara Brown, Maureen Aslin and Betsy Carey.

Includes bibliographical references.

ISBN 1-894549-23-6

1. Breast—Surgery—Popular works. 2. Chest—Surgery—Popular works. 3. Breast—Surgery—Patients—Biography. 4. Chest—Surgery—Patients— Biography. 5. Breast—Care and hygiene. I. Brown, Barbara II. Aslin, Maureen III. Carey, Betsy

RD539.8.M94 2003   618.1'9059   C2003-901593-9

Edited by Eleanor Mackay
Copyedited by Rhea Tregebov
Designed by Liz Martin
Production assistance by Beverly Deutsch

Sumach Press acknowledges the support of the Canada Council for the Arts and the Ontario Arts Council for our publishing program. We acknowledge the Government of Ontario through the Ontario Media Development Corporation's Ontario Book Initiative.

ONTARIO ARTS COUNCIL
CONSEIL DES ARTS DE L'ONTARIO

Published by
SUMACH PRESS
1415 Bathurst Street #202
Toronto, Canada
M5R 3H8

sumachpress@on.aibn.com
www.sumachpress.com

ACKNOWLEDGEMENTS

Many people have been a part of creating *My Breasts, My Choice: Journeys Through Surgery*. We especially want to thank …

Sumach Press for their commitment to publishing literature that reflects and touches women's lives. It has been a magic carpet for the project to fly on, increasing beyond measure the accessibility of *My Breasts, My Choice* for those affected by surgical intervention. Transforming *My Breasts, My Choice* into a book has been a task full of care and attention. Thank you to Beth McAuley, Lois Pike, Liz Martin, Rhea Tregebov and Eleanor Mackay from Sumach Press. Your additions, revisions and vision have been invaluable.

The Journey to Healing: Health Care section contributors — Pauline Bradbrook, Christina Strang, Jen Green, Mary Wong, Sarah Cowley, Gail Hancock, Pam Hammond, Esther Myers, Vladimir Lange, and The American Society of Plastic Surgeons — for sharing their knowledge and resources, ensuring their research is as up to date as possible, and for their willingness to make their particular health-care traditions easily available.

The ten participants — Shelley Hobbs, Kyle Scanlon, Angela, Bobbi Aubin, Nancy Viva Davis Halifax, Mirha-Soleil Ross, James Brown, Kevin, Laura and Corrin Adams — who opened their homes, their hearts, and their lives to make this book possible. Thank you.

Thanks also to those who supported the exhibit *My Breasts, My Choice: a photographic installation*.

OUR COMMUNITY SPONSOR:
The 519 Church Street Community Centre: Alison Kemper, Executive Director, The Board and Staff, particularly those directly involved in Trans Programming.

DONORS & SUPPORTERS:
Come As You Are
Toronto Women's Bookstore
AGFA
Good For Her
CPL Systems & Ken McAlpine
The Press Room
Pope Joan
Painted City Gallery
Jo-Anne Wood

Graphic Design: Linda Mayer
Exhibit Design Consultant: Michael Brisson
Media Consultant: Denny Allen
Exhibit Editing: Gillian Watts, Word Watch Editorial Services

COMMUNITY PARTNERS & RESOURCES:
Ontario Breast Cancer Community Research Initiatives
Canadian Breast Cancer Network
Harbord Health Centre
Barbara Hall
Southern Ontario Lesbian & Gays Association of Doctors (SOGLAD)
Womennet.ca

AND OUR MEDIA SPONSORS:
Xtra! Magazine
LSBNToronto.com
GayCanada.com
NOW Magazine
Siren Magazine

CONTENTS

PART II

THE JOURNEY TO HEALING

Health Care

Introduction: Beginning the Journey

Barbara Brown

In 1999, I began looking for information and images about breast surgery. I'd been thinking about breast reduction for a long time. I wanted to know what I'd look like, how it might feel, what could happen to my body, and how to heal. Surprisingly, I found very little information. What I did discover was a great interest in a resource which would both show images and tell stories. Those affected had a strong desire to share their own (their lovers', friends', mothers') experience of breast surgery. Stories began to be told and all I had to do was find a photographer ... Or so I thought. I had no idea that I was about to step into what was to become a four-year project.

My Breasts, My Choice: *a photographic installation,* which opened in October 2001 at the 519 Church Street Community Centre in Toronto, was the first expression of this project. The installation featured the photographs of ten volunteer participants who had undergone various types of breast or chest surgery. The accompanying texts were drawn from my interviews with the participants. These images and stories now also comprise "Telling Our Journeys: Personal Narratives," the first section of this book. The second section, "The Journey to Healing: Health Care," is a collection of ten articles which offer readers an accessible introduction to the procedures involved in breast and chest surgery, as well as alternative methods of self-care pre- and post-surgery.

My Breasts, My Choice would unexpectedly require much of me. Although I was and am a writer with a health-care background, I had no experience in the art world, no experience in fundraising, and little knowledge of how to get one's work into the public view. I was seduced by the energy of the idea itself and the response it was receiving. Throughout, I felt carried forward by an impetus greater than my own, an impetus I call the creative spirit meeting with a deep cultural longing.

One of the early signs of this was the response to my advertisement looking for a photographer. Knowing it was an unpaid job, sixteen people replied. Fourteen photographers later, I met Betsy Carey. Having been a photographer for almost twenty years, she brought a necessary mix of artistic experience and technical skill to the production of the exhibit and the book. But most importantly, her photography catches the essence of her subject, showing an inner-dwelling truth through the external form and image. It was clear she was the one for this project.

In the winter of 2000, Betsy and I began developing the conceptual format and started advertising for participants. In the spring of 2000, Maureen Aslin, a friend of mine and housemate of Betsy's, happened to overhear part of a planning meeting. We were feeling daunted by the scope of the work to be done and I was worried *My Breasts, My Choice* wouldn't even get off the ground. Maureen had some ideas. Her first role was in assisting with administrative coordination, to which she brought her skills in organizational process and facilitation, as well as her general ingenuity. Together, the three of us became the artistic team for *My Breasts, My Choice,* working collectively through the following year and half to mount the opening exhibit. Our aim was to explore, detail, and make accessible the realities of people's experience of breast and chest surgery, *without judgement or conclusion.* We brought a body-positive, sex-positive, pro-choice philosophical stance to our work, and a commitment to ensuring participants had full editorial say over their contribution.

Once we began interviewing, *My Breasts, My Choice* quickly became a collaborative process between the artistic team and the participants. The participants risked much of themselves and gave an immense amount of time to create this intimate and moving collection. Some were involved in a lengthy interview process; some wrote their own story. Some did both. Participants had at least one, and often two photoshoots. Some participants chose to include their full name as a part of bringing themselves and their story forward; others chose pseudonyms since their life circumstances required a greater degree of privacy. They offered their own photographs, art and poetry for use in the show. And they all played an integral role in the preparation of their texts and the choice of photographs. A central theme that became evident through the interview process was that the participants shared our desire to make information about experiences of breast and chest surgery more available. In the book, many of the participants speak of their motivation to be involved. Bobbi Aubin underwent reduction surgery as a part of a life transformation which included leaving an abusive marriage, healing from sexual abuse, and coming out as a lesbian. She

writes, "I am sharing my story for two reasons: for personal healing, and because I believe sharing life stories benefits others. I especially hope my story will help other women who are suffering."

Although the initial vision for the work was less comprehensive in terms of types of surgeries, the project came to include breast reduction surgery, gynaecomastia reduction for men, augmentation, breast cancer diagnostics, lumpectomy, mastectomy and reconstructive surgeries. Ten people — breast cancer survivors, transsexuals, and women and men choosing surgery for health or other personal reasons — came forward to share the emotional aspects of surgical intervention, relationships with health-care professionals, and their reflections on body image, self-esteem, identity and healing.

Our first interview in the fall of 2000 was with Nancy Viva Davis Halifax, a woman in her forties who, having undergone breast reduction, learned she had early stage breast cancer. Nancy elected to have a mastectomy. Nancy, Betsy and I gathered in her home for the photoshoot. With only one of us so exposed, we were doing our best to be comfortable. We chatted, put on music, lit candles, drank tea. We petted Neoka, her dog, who stayed at Nancy's side throughout. Then, with a deep breath of courage, Nancy took off her shirt. My eyes took in the small round breast, a delight to her, and the flat diagonal mastectomy scar, indicator of her unexpected discovery — the discovery that changed the direction of her life. We learned that Nancy had left her long-term employment to pursue doctoral studies in arts-informed research, which she was enrolled in at the time we met. Through her participation in *My Breasts, My Choice,* Nancy's thesis inquiry shifted and ultimately came to include the poetic transcription that she had written for the project as a primary base for her doctorate. Standing in her kitchen, awkward and half-naked, Nancy glowed.

Her passion for living was evident as she talked about the joy of having less physical pain as a result of the reduction, the struggle to come to comfort in her body, and the mix of fear and gratitude in her early discovery of cancer. Seeing her opened my vision and expanded my concept of beauty. I was blown away.

We then met Mirha-Soleil Ross, a videographer and transsexual activist who, at sixteen, in an attempt to live more successfully as a boy, had bilateral mastectomy of her naturally developing breasts. More recently, Mirha-Soleil has had breast augmentation. Her augmentation has required two surgeries thus far and a third is expected. She has no regrets. We spent much of our interview discussing the impact of second-wave feminist thought on transsexual and sex-trade worker experience and activism, a conflictual theoretical and community gap still to be bridged — something Mirha-Soleil and I unexpectedly found ourselves attempting to do in our discussion. Mirha-Soleil writes, "How condescending, demeaning it is to say that women choosing to get involved with cosmetic surgery are only doing so because of the pressure to live up to misogynistic standards of beauty. It is denying us any wisdom and agency in the decisions we make about our bodies and lives."

Throughout the interview process, something inside me, something different with each person, was required to crack open. When we began, I naively imagined we'd hear simple stories of breast surgery, the ins and outs of surgical intervention, perhaps discover some "helpful hints." However, there are no simple stories when it comes to our bodies, our decisions, our souls, our lives. Each participant that we met challenged us to think and feel and look deeper, more broadly, more comprehensively. For example, early in the interviewing process, someone idly asked, "Why not have male participants, as well as women and trans?" After talking and thinking about it as a team, we said, "Yes. Let's do it." — which ultimately made it possible for Kyle Scanlon to participate. Kyle comments that his choice for involvement as a transsexual man was made possible by the fact that biological men were also welcome as participants.

However, by including men, questions regarding the implications of the project's title and the power of language to include or exclude were highlighted — the word "breast" was not one that the men identified with. Two of the men in the project, Kyle and James Brown, speak openly about the process of transitioning from female to male. They emphasize the importance of speaking about the creation of their chests, not the removal of their breasts. Each followed a different path for transition, James through a gender identity disorder clinic, and Kyle independent of such a program. The supports they received medically for their surgeries varied substantially (both had two surgeries), as did their experiences in negotiating a medical system not familiar with transsexual experience. Kevin, the third male in the project, describes his attempt to access surgical intervention for the development of breast tissue (gynaecomastia), a result of prescribed liver medications. As Kevin writes, "I tried to correct a wrong — or correct something that made me uncomfortable — and I got butchered." All three men, as with many of the participants, struggled with the financial weight of repeated surgical intervention.

Questions about the book's title were also raised by some breast cancer survivors who did not experience their diagnostic procedures or surgery as a "choice." Shelley Hobbs and Angela each faced a possible diagnosis of breast cancer. Both felt the life-altering fear that comes when waiting for such results. "My world came to a screeching halt at that word: MALIGNANCY. It echoed through me like a harsh shattering of glass in the belly of a cave," Shelley writes of hearing her breast cancer diagnosis. Angela's tests proved to be negative. She reflects, "… the fear of having breast cancer brought me back to the preciousness of life. I want to continue to live and celebrate my life in this awareness. I chose to be a part of this project because being photographed is about bringing my breasts into the light." Although their outcomes were radically different, neither experienced a sense of choice in the procedures required, and for both, room for decision-making was limited. Pauline Bradbrook discusses the experience of having had "no choice" regarding her own mastectomy in her chapter on peer support, which is included in the second section of this book.

Corrin Adams and Laura each made very conscious choices about their surgeries, with differing impacts. Laura was in the midst of divorcing her husband, grieving her mother's death, and addressing the costs of alcoholism and familial violence that she had experienced as a child. In the midst of this she decided to pursue a long-time dream of having breast augmentation. She writes, "The augmentation represented taking back many things, including making a decision solely based on me … Now I don't even think about the implants, they're so congruent with my body. I would miss them terribly if for some medical reason I was told I shouldn't have them in."

At age sixteen, seeking what she then saw as freedom in her body and movement, freedom from the ways feminine sexuality is culturally constructed and limiting, Corrin chose breast reduction. She made the decision without substantial medical information or personal support. Corrin writes, "My desire for the longest time — for years, for years — was wishing that I had not made that decision at all, wishing I could have my breasts back. Why? Because I didn't want to have the scars. I didn't want the responsibility. It was a desire for a return to my natural, untouched state. I felt like I had betrayed the whole woman race." After many years of living through those emotions and

beliefs, Corrin now feels differently: "'This is my body. This *is* my body.' That's profound for me. It's the difference between this being my body in its unnatural form — which is how I thought of it, me being separate from my body — and realizing that my body is an expression of who I am and where I've been." Both Laura and Corrin found their way to a place of integration and acceptance of their choices, although with radically different paths. Their stories bring to the forefront the importance of cultural context, self-awareness, support and access to information for fully informed decision-making. They also highlight how our systems do and do not provide those facing surgery with these components.

The articles in the second section of this book, "The Journey to Healing: Health Care," were developed specifically to address the type of concerns Corrin and others had raised. Participants and viewers of the exhibit frequently commented on the dearth of accessible resources available to those facing surgery. Indeed, it was the absence of such resources in my own search that had initiated the project. We hope that this section will also be beneficial in broadening health-care professionals' awareness of pre- and post-surgical interventions available for surgery patients. In approaching the "The Journey to Healing," as in the rest of the project, we strove to maintain a holistic perspective on health and personhood. Pauline Bradbrook and Christina Strang write on models of empowerment through social support, access to information and advocacy; Jen Green details specific nutritional and naturopathic interventions for breast health and pre- and post-operative care. Mary Wong reviews the Traditional Chinese Medicine approach to our bodies' energy system and the response to surgical intervention. Dr. Vladimir Lange and the American Society of Plastic Surgeons provide detailed information regarding the actual surgical procedures. Sarah Cowley, Gail

Hancock and Pam Hammond write on the benefits of Swedish massage, lymphatic drainage massage, and hydrotherapy for clients pre- and post-operatively. Esther Myers discusses the overall healing capacity of yoga and outlines basic exercises helpful post-operatively. These chapters are followed with a brief bibliography of print and on-line resources. As with the voices of the participants, we have attempted to make room for a broad range of perspectives regarding health and well-being. Far from being comprehensive, the health-care chapters act as a compendium of resources from which further research can be done.

All these conversations and considerations infused the creative process and raised the question of how, or even whether, our health-care system and professionals, the art world, or social support services might allow themselves to be broken open by such complexities. During the first year there was clearly interest within the general public — participants were coming forward, Betsy and I were doing interviews and photo-shoots — but our funding and administrative work was not moving ahead as readily. Crossing boundaries of art, health care, and sociological grouping, a primary strength of *My Breasts, My Choice*, actually created roadblocks in our attempts to secure funding and support. We didn't fit into any of the neat categories created by art councils, health-care research, or affected community groups. The 519 Church Street Community Centre came on in the midst of this, joining us in November 2000. The 519 provided us a home base to work from and a structural presence in the world. Becoming involved with *My Breasts, My Choice* as a community sponsor launched the 519 in their involvement in arts programming. Having a community sponsor and administrative assistance propelled us into our next step, which was raising funds to cover the costs of production. By hosting "Skin Deep: A Silent Auction," Betsy's series of double-exposure photographs, and by mounting a mail request fundraising effort, we were able to provide a modest financial base to buy materials and advertise. The work continued.

Over the next year Betsy, Maureen and I produced what became *My Breasts, My Choice: a photographic installation*. Through preparation of the exhibit, we learned about graphic design, publicity, and the nuts-and-bolts of exhibit materials. Maureen's research skills and artistic understanding were key during this time. Stepping beyond the administrative support she had been providing, she became our exhibit design coordinator. In the summer of 2001 we began conversations with Sumach Press. Their immediate interest in the project as a book provided increased momentum.

There are many without whom *My Breasts, My Choice* would never have found its way to fruition. The support of gutsy, caring individuals and companies, as well as organizations involved in breast cancer and transsexual support, has enabled *My Breasts, My Choice* to become a reality. I say "gutsy" because the project intentionally crosses culturally established boundaries of identities relating to breast and chest surgery. To stand with this diversity of affected peoples takes courage. In connecting with so many supportive people, there was one particular exchange that stirred a question worth noting here. We met Michael Brisson, architect and design consultant, when he called seeking information regarding the influence on breast surgery procedures of a cultural preference for a "natural aesthetic." He wondered, from a modern art perspective, if there were other ways to perform these surgeries that incorporated the scarring as a feature, rather than trying to hide or minimize them. His question remains unanswered.

As the launch neared, there was for me a pervading sense of having to let go. I suspect many artists face this same moment. *My Breasts, My Choice: a photographic installation* had to stand on its own. In October 2001, the exhibit opened at the 519 Church Street Community Centre. The show was organized with Breast Cancer Awareness Month activities. It was an exhilarating time. This was my first public work of art, and not only was it being incredibly well received, it was touching people's lives.

There are some gaps in the work that as a team we regret. A primary one is that none of the participants have had a "tramflap" reconstructive surgery, one of the most common breast reconstructive procedures. As well, the number of people of colour involved is small, only two participants, and none of the participants are over the age of sixty. Our original goal for participants was twelve, however the book has only ten. This is because as a team we were committed to holding open the last two spots for older people, those of colour, and someone who had had a tramflap. Despite an extensive second round of advertising for participants, no one came forward within the production time frame. In the screening process, there were people that fit into these categories, however for many reasons, including family pressure, their own time constraints, discomfort with being photographed, and cultural prohibitions, they had to step out of the project. Through the exhibit, we have since met many others who are eager to tell their stories. Unfortunately, we have not been able to include them here. Our intent was to also include a chapter on aboriginal teaching and healing. During the production phase of the book, two confirmed writers had to step out of the work due to life circumstances. Ultimately, we ran out of time to secure a contributor. Potential contributors discussed the limited number of aboriginal people accessing cosmetic surgery due to economic constraints, and mentioned that the incidence of breast cancer is small in comparison to other health concerns within aboriginal communities. Given

the imbalance in participation in relation to racial diversity, we are left with questions of potential cultural bias within the project's format itself, as well as larger questions of societal racial and economic biases regarding these surgeries. We invite discussion and feedback regarding these unanswered questions as a part of *My Breasts, My Choice*'s ongoing dialogue with viewers and readers.

My Breasts, My Choice: Journeys Through Surgery is rooted in the tradition of storytelling, in the process of knowing through seeing, and in relationships of willingness, courage and trust. Respect for the telling of the stories and for the exposure of self through images was paramount in the preparation of *My Breasts, My Choice* as an exhibit and book. Throughout, we sought a truthful reflection of those participating so that those involved might, in the process, see and hear themselves. This commitment was woven into our creative process, our philosophical stance, and our hopes for the project. In the preparation of *My Breasts, My Choice,* the artistic team of Betsy Carey, photographer, Maureen Aslin, exhibit design coordinator, and myself, Barbara Brown, interviewer and editor, founded our work on the hope that this project would provoke thought and dialogue about the sociological, political and personal implications of breast and chest surgery. *My Breasts, My Choice* is designed to be a tool for information, education and support for people facing surgery, those close to them, and health-care professionals. We encourage you develop a forum to hear more of these stories and to continue stepping across arbitrary divisions. We hope you will use this book as a springboard for further reflection, and for personal and social change. We believe that each person's story has a unique contribution and that, combined, the strength of the stories is multiplied. We were able to bring forward ten people's stories although we know there are many, many others.

For me, with each step in the process, with the meeting of every person involved, I have been touched and changed. The participants invited us in to their intimate places. For that, I am grateful. I am still sitting with my initial question about my own breast surgery, but I am clearer, more prepared, and ready to wait until I know for sure what it is I want to do. I am radically different for having been a part of this project. And yet, as my own particular story comes to an end, even in being different I am left with a kernel of desire that is similar to that with which I began the process. If my dream for this project came true, it would be that in reading *My Breasts, My Choice: Journeys Through Surgery* you are encouraged to somewhere, anywhere, tell your own story.

My Breasts, My Choice has been a tremendous vehicle for my own learning and personal reflection. Both the stories of the participants and the collaborative creative process have deeply changed my life.

MAUREEN ASLIN
Exhibit Design Coordinator

It was an honour to document these profoundly moving experiences. I greatly admire the participants' courage and dignity.

BETSY CAREY
Photographer

PART I

TELLING OUR JOURNEYS
Personal Narratives

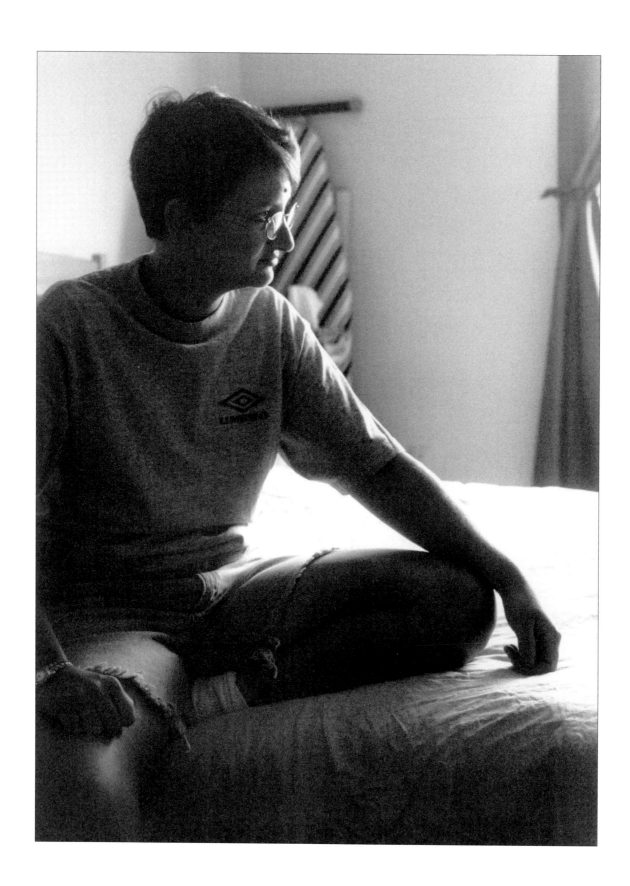

SHELLEY HOBBS
A Tale of Two Boobs

Shelley Hobbs is a breast cancer survivor who had a double mastectomy with implant reconstruction. As a child, Shelley battled with cancer of the kidney, then metastatic lung cancer. Just before her fortieth birthday, she received a diagnosis of bilateral breast cancer. Shelley speaks of living with the fear of "IT" (cancer) returning all her life, and with this diagnosis she was required to face that fear directly.

Shelley views coming out and telling her story as a breast cancer survivor equal in importance to coming out as a lesbian. This perspective is what encouraged her to participate in the photo exhibit of My Breasts, My Choice *and in this book. Shelley works as a lawyer for a government agency providing advocacy on behalf of incapable adults, those at personal and/or financial risk. She is also a sports (especially hockey) fanatic, dog lover and writer.*

When I was six years old, I was diagnosed with a Wilm's tumour on my left kidney. I had emergency surgery to remove my kidney and other assorted bits of affected plumbing. When I was seven, I had surgery on a metastatic lung tumour for which I had to go to Winnipeg. My family lived in Thunder Bay at the time. I lost about half of my right lung in the second surgery. I had another lung tumour when I was ten, which was irradiated. I spent my childhood in and out of hospital and on and off chemotherapy and radiation until I was pronounced cured at age twelve. The scars I carried, along with an underdeveloped torso and a slight scoliosis of the spine undoubtedly affected my self-image over the years.

Since I was a rambunctious kid, my chest was not much of an issue until puberty arrived, when in fact I was more embarrassed about having tiny breasts than by my surgical scars. Fortunately, by the time I'd reached adulthood, I had other things to worry about, notably coming out as a lesbian and, in the fall of 1980, escaping at nineteen to university in Toronto. I am also congenitally hearing impaired. I use a hearing aid and miss half of what's said in movies. I speak some American Sign Language, but I'm not fluent.

But I digress. This is, after all, the tale of two boobs.

As I ambled towards my fortieth birthday, my personal situation was good. I had been single for a few years after having been in a series of monogamous relationships for most of my twenties and thirties, and having had the odd fling here and there. I had a job I love: I am a lawyer for a government agency that advocates on behalf of mentally incapable adults who are at serious risk of personal or financial harm.

By April 2001, I had accomplished my modest goals of acquiring a new couch, a new car, and a condo before reaching the big 4-0. I had completed my second season of learning to play hockey and had scored my first goal ever. Despite a continual pining for love, a girlfriend, or at least — okay, who are we kidding? — sex, I was reasonably happy.

Then, a few months before turning forty, came ... the Finding of the Lump. Dr. Susan Love is an American breast health guru. She takes the position that women should do regular breast self-exams, not in anticipation of our bodies betraying us, but rather to get to know our own bodies and breasts so that we might notice anything different or unusual. I agree. Knowing my own body — physically, physiologically, and sexually — was very much the key.

I found the Lump in mid-April 2001. This was right before the closing date on my condo, as well as the ten-day holiday in Wales and England I had planned for the beginning of May. I made an appointment with my general practitioner for April 30. My GP was on maternity leave, however, so I met her locum, a young doctor who looked as though she'd graduated *very* recently. Once I had stripped down, she looked at my body and exclaimed, "My god, you've had surgery!"

No kidding, I thought, but more kindly replied, "Didn't you read my chart?"

"Oh, no," she said, "I like to be surprised."

She asked if I was premenstrual and when my last period had been. Then she did a breast exam while standing as far away as she could get. I wondered if she was perturbed by the word "lesbian" written at the top of the information sheet with my chart. Maybe it was the fact that she had expected to treat nothing more than runny noses and babies, and instead got a potential "big C."

I joked about how odd it was, not knowing each other from a hole in the ground and having to do this exam, but she just kept muttering about my period. I told her I was not premenstrual and that this lump was not normal for me. I asked to have an ultrasound done and she filled out the appropriate form. When I called

the ultrasound clinic, the receptionist said she'd squeeze me in the next day.

A pleasant female technician performed the ultrasound. For several minutes she was chatty and then all expression vanished from her face. She finished, gave me paper towels to wipe up the blue goop, and said I'd need a mammogram.

"Okay," I said, "Could we make an appointment after my holidays?"

"No," she said. "You're having one right now."

Oh.

So, on to the mammogram. I had never had one before. The mammogram technician, who was also very kind, looked like she was going to give herself a back cramp trying to mash my teeny-tiny boobs in between the acrylic plates. I have always had great nipples, but no breasts of any note. I haven't worn a bra since I was sixteen. Even when I was PMSing, I barely jiggled. The poor technician shoved and arranged and flattened as best she could, somehow managing to get the necessary images.

She looked at the film and then left the room. Before leaving she told me not to change. I huddled on a chair in that ridiculous thin blue cotton shift wishing there was a magazine in the room. Instead I only had information posters showing women who actually had boobs, and how the mammogram compressed them into pancakes from every angle, to stare at. Ow, I thought sympathetically.

On her return, the technician said, "You'll need a fine-needle biopsy."

"Fine," I replied. "Can we set up the appointment for after my holiday?"

"No," she said. "We're doing it now."

Oh.

I moved to a third room in which there was another ultrasound machine. The radiologist in charge, a woman, and a male technologist entered and began the procedure. A fine-needle biopsy consists of inserting a long, thin needle without a local anaesthetic into the lump or area of concern in the breast. Fluid and cells from the area are sucked into the syringe and sent to the pathology lab for testing.

"Well," I told the fellow, "you probably won't believe this, but you're the first man to touch my breasts since I was a teenager." It took a minute for the penny to drop, and then he laughed, having spied the beaded rainbow bracelet on my left wrist.

"You've got great pectoral muscles," he said pleasantly, as he jabbed about.

"Thanks," I said. "I work out when I can."

I thanked them both for their help and the speed with which they had done the tests. "I am off on holidays now," I declared.

The radiologist took my hand and told me in a gentle Voice of Doom, "Have a lovely holiday, dear, and don't worry about a thing."

I smiled, and thought, Great ... *I'm gonna die!*

I walked back to the tiny change booth, drew the curtains, and tears burned my eyes. I couldn't tell if I felt terror or sadness or outrage. It all felt surreal.

I don't remember how I got home. I don't remember if I talked to anyone. I only remember that when I got there, I roused my dog from her nap and hugged her.

I had lived with the possibility of IT returning since I was in Grade One. IT is cancer. I had fought against the insidious effects from anxiety about IT every time I laced up my cleats or stripped down in a communal shower or argued against unfairness. ITs return this time felt so fast and so sudden that, once I heard the gentle kindness in the radiologist's voice, I knew — with absolute certainty — IT was in both breasts.

There have been very few moments in which I have felt my reality change, my life alter utterly, my essential self both threatened and established, all in one short moment. This was one of them.

I went on my holiday. I wandered by myself through north Wales and then London, thinking about who would look after my dog, feeling depressed because I hadn't finished any writing, imagining I'd just drop out of existence on this planet without so much as a ripple. Death and disfigurement permeated my thoughts. I spent much of my time in transit, sitting waiting for buses or trains, and the rest of my time milling about with other tourists. It was a struggle to pay attention to the experience. Despite having looked forward to this journey for years, I felt disconnected from the event, as though I were watching someone else shuffle through the castles and museums and crowds.

There is an odd little station on the main line into and out of northwest Wales called Dovey Junction. It consists of a cement platform on which one light standard and a phone booth stand naked in the middle of acres of rolling sheep country. The nearest building is a crumbling castle a mile away on a hill. The nearest road runs alongside that castle. It looks like something from *Dr. Who*. It was set up as a transfer station for passengers, so that the train would not have to be re-routed. Therefore it stood in the middle of nowhere. I felt as if the train schedule had been deemed more important than had the passengers themselves.

After the Finding and the Tests, I took a trip to a portable Dovey Junction inside myself. I felt the same isolation I'd felt at the real junction, the same emptiness as I waited under a hard grey sky — waiting for a train, waiting. I felt the same loneliness, insignificance in a disinterested patch of a foreign land. I remember feeling as though I'd been placed outside the rest of humanity, deemed inconvenient almost, because of my necessary choice of destination. My destination had been a specific town, and because of that, I'd had to disembark at Dovey Junction and wait for another train to take me there. It's a good thing I took pictures and made notes during my trip; otherwise, I doubt I would have remembered any of it except for this isolation.

When I got back, I saw the locum physician again on May 22. She seemed unable to cope. I told her just to hand over the results from the ultrasound and mammogram so I could read them myself. In full caps, lest one miss their significance, the results were stated in these words:

IN THE LEFT BREAST ... THERE IS A 9 MM SOLID LESION NOTED LATERALLY AT THREE O'CLOCK ... IN THE RIGHT BREAST, THERE IS A MALIGNANT-TYPE CLUSTER OF CALCIFICATIONS ... BOTH OF THE ABOVE LESIONS ARE SUSPICIOUS FOR MALIGNANCY.

My world came to a screeching halt at that word: *MALIGNANCY*. It echoed through me like a harsh shattering of glass in the belly of a cave.

If you have ever thought you had experienced loneliness before, it is nothing compared to the alienation that word malignancy brings to you. You are so alone. Nobody goes down that cold hallway but you; nobody goes into surgery but you; only you wake up to whatever has been done to you. I had felt this loneliness before, long ago, as a child. Now I was abruptly back in that place.

Next stop, May 28: the oncology surgeon. It turns out that she trained under the oncologist/haemotologist who treated me ages ago but who is now retired. It felt like old home week.

She had the fine-needle biopsy results, which confirmed malignancy on the right and "highly suspicious" on the left. "I see," I replied. "So we're looking at at least one mastectomy?"

"Yes. But first, we need core biopsies to confirm the nature of the malignancy, especially whether or not it is invasive."

On the way home, I purchased *Dr. Susan Love's Breast Book* and a Canadian book, *Breast Cancer,* by Olivotto, Gelmon, and Kuusk. I devoured them. Then I rummaged on the Internet.

It was with the quiet turning of pages that I truly fathomed that I would have to have my breasts removed. Both of them, if I wanted to be certain.

I learned that calcifications are tiny pockets of calcium deposited in places where cancer cells have sucked up all the nutrients and killed the surrounding normal cells. They appear like patches of buckshot — unlike a tumour, which is a solid chunk of cancer. Sometimes, however, the ultrasound pictures do not tell the radiologist whether or not a solid object is cancer. Sometimes the biopsies do not even reveal the nature of all the cells extracted. Sometimes the surgeon actually has to cut a large piece out of the suspicious area for testing. This is called a surgical biopsy. If the lump is small enough, the surgeon might cut out the entire lump or tumour but leave the rest of the breast; this is called a lumpectomy. Lumpectomies are often followed up with radiation treatments to ensure the elimination of any stray cancer cells outside the tumour site.

I learned that forty is the usual age for women who were irradiated for childhood cancers to develop breast cancer. Funny, none of my GPs ever mentioned this likelihood to me. My childhood radiation treatments also meant that I was not a candidate for a lumpectomy, as further radiation to the places where I'd already received it might cause more cancer to develop.

My breasts didn't hurt. There was no discharge, no redness or funny patches of skin. They were, with the exception of the Lump, as they always had been.

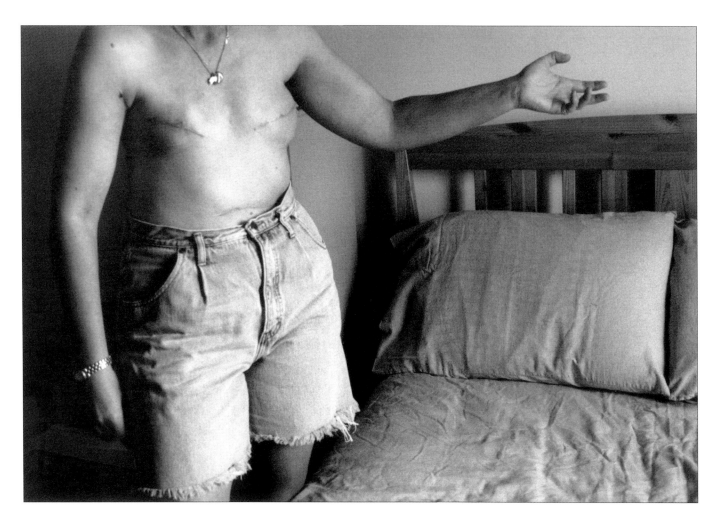

The nipples still worked; they were still connected directly to my clitoris. I closed my eyes and remembered the last time I'd had sex. 'Twas at the Pussy Palace, a women's bathhouse. My first time there. It was a frolic, a dance, a giggle, an odd mix of Girl Guide camp and Sluts-R-Us. I ran around naked — scars, tiny boobs and all — and had a marvellous time.

Gone.

As I waited to have the core biopsy done, going through a time of turning over ideas, of making cups of coffee, of stroking my dog, I realized that *they* were back in my life. *They* wanted another pound of flesh — probably about one and a half pounds, if pushed. *They* had come for another instalment in the payment plan for my life. Amongst the archetypes I'd created as a child, *they* are the people who wield the knives and the needles and the platitudes. *They* are the doctors, the nurses, the specialists, and *they* were challenging me again.

Goddammit! These breasts might not be perfect, but they are mine!

My breasts had given me — and some other love-ly women — great pleasure over the years. My breasts were integral to my sexuality. I was suddenly posses-sive of them. My hindbrain did not want to listen to my forebrain talk about life and death. When I was a kid, my parents had always played a trump card. If I was angry or wanted to complain or did not want to be "brave" or to be on display to interns or submit to tests, my parents would tell me, "They are saving your life, dear." Put up with it, don't question it; even if it hurts or is embarrassing; you must be grateful to *them*. *They* had all the power and I had none. Not even over my own bodily functions.

They were back. IT was back. I was enraged. I was at Dovey Junction and *they* were waiting at every sta-tion I could go to from there. I had no escape route. *They* would find me. IT would find me. I, who prided myself on my independence, who had ended an abu-sive relationship, who had fought clinical depression and won, who had a good job and supportive family and friends, who *loved* life, was now back where I had started: where IT had control, where everything was orchestrated by *them*, the gowned and chemical-smelling saviours.

If you want to gut someone of their self-esteem or nullify their sense of existence, let alone importance, take away their ability to decide, their control over themselves. Make them dependent. Take away their ability to choose.

"I am an adult now," I declared to myself. "I will choose what I want to do." I asked the oncology sur-geon for a referral to a plastic surgeon. My first meet-ing with him was set for June 6.

I went back to talk to the oncology surgeon. She advised that if I wanted reconstruction, the bilateral mastectomy would have to be scheduled for a day when the plastic surgeon was also available. It could be as soon as a week or as long a wait as three weeks; it would be cancelled if I got a cold or had an injury. Any delay could bump me into danger, could mean months of waiting while IT grew inside me.

I cancelled soccer for the duration. I'd played with the same team since 1989, but this year they'd have to find another goalie. I had signed up for summer hock-ey, but that was out as well. My main source of thera-py, sports, was now not available. I resolved to keep fit somehow. My dog would get a lot of walks.

The clinic set June 20 as a day for post-operative tests, bone scans, a liver ultrasound, and an x-ray, on the assumption that I'd have had my surgery by then. Those tests checked for the spread of cancer around the breast area.

I couldn't help but think of another bad M-word: metastasis. Further dalliance with portents of doom. More waiting. During the bone scan, as my skeleton coalesced into sparkles on a television screen, the male technologist, looking at my rainbow bracelet, asked matter-of-factly if I played golf. "Did you know you only have one kidney?" he inquired.

It was a miracle, really, that I went so quickly through the quantity of tests I needed to. The entire experience became a pointed reminder for me of the effects of privilege — my privilege. I am white, I have a well-paying job with good benefits, and I am blessed with supportive family and friends.

What if I were mentally impaired, not fluent in English, without benefits or sick leave, unemployed, family- and friendless, a refugee, a single parent, transgendered, elderly, physically disabled, or had religious or cultural imperatives that conflicted with the standard medical methods ... What then?

I met with the plastic surgeon, a young, happening

kind of guy. I nicknamed him "the Boob Dude." He surveyed my body, poked here and there. "Good pliable skin," he said. "We can't do the tramflap because you're too thin and the surgery on your abdomen has compromised your belly area, but we can do saline silicone implants." I was flushed with relief. I was eligible for artificial breasts of some kind. I was surprised by how much I wanted to wake up with something, even implants.

"It's covered by OHIP," said the Dude. "I can make you fake nipples with tattooed colouring after your breast mounds and implants settle into position." The Boob Dude was brief but cheerful. He seemed competent. I had to trust him; if I waited to get a second opinion, it would mean Delay. What he said matched what I had read, so I decided to proceed. The new boobs wouldn't be real, but they would be better than nothing.

I was already a freak. I couldn't bear the thought of more mutilation. My whole life had been spent as an alien: scars, queer, hearing loss, too smart for my own good. If *they* were going to chop off my breasts, I wanted something to take their place, fake or not. Better than barren skin and ribs and muscle.

Next, I had the core biopsies. In this procedure, the technician injected my breasts with local anaesthetic and then, using ultrasound to assist with positioning, inserted a large needle shaped like a medieval lancet with jaws into the area of the Lump and the calcifications. With a loud cracking sound, the lancet snapped up a chunk of flesh and off to the pathology lab the samples went.

I imagined my file growing steadily and relentlessly, each piece of paper adding another aspect of my most intimate self to the binder. It all seemed so mechanical.

I found I was gradually dissociating myself from my own body, from my own breasts. It was as if they were family members who were moving away forever, and I wanted to ease the pain by drawing back from them before they left.

Throughout those two months of waiting for a surgery date and undergoing other preparatory medical procedures, I remained active in the world.

How do people tolerate six- and eight-month waiting periods when they know they have something growing inside them, draining them, trying to kill them? What happens to them when they're held out over the void for so long?

I attended Gay Pride Dyke March marshal training, as well as my friends Linda and Caroline's baby shower. I umpired a softball game. I worked, attended court, drafted pleadings, and negotiated outcomes. Hell, I even organized an obligatory department open house. I flailed away at a golf tournament — ironically, to raise funds for breast cancer research. I helped coach my soccer team.

But I also found myself sitting and staring. Empty. Shocked. I made arrangements for my dog's care, signed a power of attorney, wrote a holograph will. My work colleagues quietly began taking over my practice, including my most difficult cases. They did this even though we didn't have enough lawyers, even though their own practices were jam-packed. They stepped in, and I will never be able to thank them enough.

I moved into my condo on May 26. I packed, switched my utilities, redirected my mail, dumped old, broken furniture, and sent out new address cards — I was busy, and it was less stressful than I thought it might be. I thought, My nerve endings are numb.

My dog, Digby, was a constant source of renewal and joy. She spent almost every night curled up against the small of my back.

I dealt with frantic parents, my fabulously supportive and beloved brother and sister-in-law, my wonderful chosen family of friends, ex-lovers and biological family members. I needed comfort and, equally, I needed to be left alone. I was a piece of rope stretched so tight across a chasm that the slightest breeze made it hum. I was exhausted, yet could not sleep. I found myself deliberately not touching my breasts.

Sorry, Dr. Love, it does feel like a betrayal. But by whom? My own flesh? Them? The Goddess?

It had been just one month since the mammogram. It might as well have been a decade. The surgeon informed me of the core biopsy results: invasive carcinoma on one side and fragments of papillary lesion, atypical, on the other.

Apparently the cell structure morphology was "suggestive of invasive lobular carcinoma with 90 percent of the tumour cells positive for estrogen receptors and 70 percent positive for progesterone receptors." No one had asked the pathologist to test for the latter; the lab usually tests for progesterone receptors after surgery. It was kind of the technician to have made the extra effort. It meant that I would be a good candidate for the newest treatment with tamoxifen, and it saved me time; I didn't have to wait for my oncologist's request for the testing.

I told my oncologist that I wanted the implants and that I had decided I wanted both breasts to come off. Even though we didn't know for sure about the papillary lesion, with my history of radiation treatments, it was likely that anything peculiar that was not yet cancer would become cancer. Also, the insertion of the implants would be more effective if both were done at the same time.

I would be having a prophylactic mastectomy —

an odd term that makes me laugh. Prophylactic: an old term for a condom, the prevention of birth. In this case, it would be the prevention of my death. Or so I hoped. I don't know what the surgeon hoped for. She displayed a professional detachment, a determined non-involvement. She was not mean or uncaring; I believe she behaved in this way simply because she had a shitty job. As time went by, she did warm to me a bit.

A date for surgery was proposed, an opening created by a cancellation.

Who is that other woman, and why was her surgery cancelled? I sent out a hug through the ether to wherever she was.

The date was for the day after my fortieth birthday, if the Boob Dude could fit me into his schedule.

It meant I'd miss Gay Pride Week. I haven't missed Pride since 1981. I e-mailed the committee chairpeople to say I might not be there for my annual volunteering activity. Somewhere far, far away I had in my mind some silly idea of a big 4-0 party. Maybe later. In the end Boob Dude turned out to be unavailable, and I was glad, as I hadn't set up dog-sitting and post-surgery care with my friends and kin.

I went to Pride and tasted it as though it would be my last. I chatted up young women and flirted mildly with old chums. I herded happy lesbians on Dyke Day and manoeuvred thousands into position on the day of the Pride March. There were pipe bands, floats with buff guys, "Bears," flag twirlers, semi-naked leather gals, Dykes on Bikes, children, music and dancing. The Pride marshals wore cowboy hats with sheriff's stars. We looked appropriately ridiculous, and I knew it was the best Pride there had been in years.

The next date selected for surgery was July 11, 2001. By this time I had my support in place: old

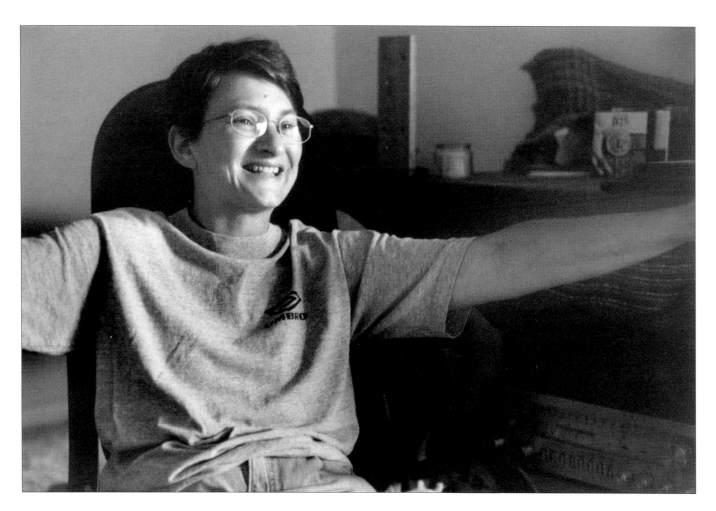

friends, chosen family, parents to do dog care. I decided to take a couple of pictures of my breasts using the bathroom mirror and a self-timer. I knew I would want to know, years later, what they used to look like. Maybe I could make a boob memorial plaque. I could hang it up next to my O'Keeffe vagina-flower print.

When the surgery took place it seemed as though it happened around me rather than *to* me. I had a left simple mastectomy and a right modified radical mastectomy. Both breasts and nipples were removed and some of my right lymph nodes were taken out. The surgeon placed the saline implants — silicone baggies filled with salt water — against my ribs behind my pectoral muscles to create the breast mounds. Drains were inserted under both arms. A fastidious soul, I had to learn to cope with dressings and drainage. The drains came out after about a week.

My stay in the hospital lasted for two and a half days. They had originally scheduled me to go home after less than twenty-four hours, but once I was actually in a ward bed, the time could be extended "if necessary."

What if I had had no home to go to? What if I had no one to argue on my behalf that it was too soon to send me out into the world?

The physiotherapist showed me exercises to do after the surgery to ensure that I would restore "full range of movement." I thought the women in the exercise drawings looked absurdly serene as they wall-crawled and rotated and slept demurely on their artfully arranged pillows. Have you ever tried to sleep with both arms elevated over your heart? I know I looked neither demure nor serene. I cursed like a sailor.

As a result of the surgery, I will have permanent numbness in my armpits and on the underside of my right arm where the lymph nodes were removed. I will also have permanent numbness around the scars, which run horizontally across my chest. Once when the nurse checked my dressings I snuck a look at my breasts. It was weird to see them with no nipples. My new nipples would also be without sensation.

Over the next four weeks, I did not show anyone my chest except the visiting nurse who changed the dressings, and Boob Dude, who was relentlessly upbeat. Occasionally, I showed my breasts to my friend who is a nurse. Under a t-shirt they look almost even. In a swimming pool, my breasts actually bobbed! They never did that before! I was quick to claim the implants as my new breasts. Although still mindful of their deceit — those baggies beneath my pecs — I felt grateful that when I applied vitamin E cream or when I saw them in the shower, these breasts looked round and substantial — abnormal, peculiar, but substantial.

It is still terrifying for me to think about a non-clinical viewing. To think of ever dropping my clothes on the floor in front of a potential sex partner is overwhelming. I, who have always been a nudie, who would bring a lover breakfast in bed wearing nothing

but a smile, am now fighting the gentle suggestions of well-meaning friends that I should "just wear a nice camisole." "Hide them," is what I hear. "If they are ugly, just hide them."

For the rest of my life? A cutesy effing camisole, a piece of fabric between me and the universe . . . forever? The suggestion is abhorrent to me. Dishonest. It makes me think of people who ask, "Gee, do you tell everyone you're a lesbian?" Yes, I do. I believe it is my duty to be out, if only for those who cannot be. Is it my duty to expose my surgery for the same reason? If I cannot trust my skin to human exposure, especially to someone whose own skin I will want to see and touch and taste, how am I to live? Skulking? Are these new breasts going to make me give up the acceptance of self, warts and all, that I have fought so hard to achieve?

Yet they are ugly. They're funny-looking. Maybe the Boob Dude can do realistic-looking nipples, but the scars will remain. The implants will continue to look peculiar. My friends have been supportive. "Hey," they've said, "You have the firmest breasts of any forty-year-old I know." "You could get a nipple ring and it won't hurt." Or "Creative tattooing, eh? Zebra stripes or colours?"

My breasts look okay under a sports bra.

Does the fact that the coverage is sports-related, a part of my usual identity, make this kind of coverage more palatable?

I have been off work now for the longest period in my life, and am only slowly finding the energy to write again. I have gradually begun to regain my cardiovascular conditioning, I am doing my physiotherapy exercises — things that a sports person understands are important. However, I can't imagine showing off these scars the way I might compare my knee surgery scar with those of my friends'.

And, at some point, I have to return to the Big Issue for me. Sex. The first point of contact with a woman's body after kissing her lips is often the touch of her breasts, her nipples. My nipples though, even after the Boob Dude's finest efforts, will not be responsive. I won't feel someone touching me there.

What do other women who have implants think and feel? They must have made the same compromise: looks over sensation. How do they feel about that decision? How do I feel about that decision? I am grateful for my life, but does that preclude me mourning this loss?

"Well," as my friend the nurse says, "You still have your 'down there'!" It's a good thing I'm experienced in bed, and that I've learned to be good with toys and tools. Maybe, if I'm good enough, the gal won't give a shit that I have weird boobs. Maybe.

My choice to have both breasts removed turned out to be a good one. Both had cancer. One was malignant and invasive, the other *in situ,* which means cancerous but not growing. Most likely the swift response has stopped all the cancer in its tracks. As I mourn for my old breasts and adjust to the new, I am reassured that my choice was the right one for me. Still, I am afraid. IT may not be vanquished, and *they* may return at any time. I live knowing this.

Now, I have a choice about how to live. As a child in the hospital, I learned to count my blessings on a regular basis. I learned how to be patient, especially with others. I learned how to wait. I ultimately learned how to see *them* as people, to forgive their actions, and especially their inaction. I learned to value having even small choices, such as what to have for breakfast or what clothes to wear that day or what book to read.

As I have often told my clients, who are people with very few opportunities to make choices in their lives, they can always say, "I don't have to like this!"

Every decision that I make is a step towards establishing greater power in my own self. It is something I can take with me anywhere, no matter what happens. I have decided to get a new puppy, a baby brother for Digby. I have decided to play hockey again, even though I have to wear extra gear because my arms will bruise easily. I have decided that, despite my fears, I will write this story and have these photographs taken. I think of it this way: somewhere there is someone else who is also afraid, who is feeling alone. That ends when we talk to each other.

UPDATES:
One Year Later

One year later, much has happened. I played hockey as a winger and was voted the "most improved" player on my team for this season. Digby's baby brother, Cooper, was born four days after my surgery and is a delight. Just before Pride Weekend, 2002, I was blessed with a new gal in my life, a loving, kind, very sexual woman with whom I have been naked *and* crazy. (Bless you, Joan!) And in November, 2002, I won a gold medal with my fast pitch softball team at the Sydney Gay Games.

Two Years Later

In February of 2003, I had the implants removed due to complications from my history of radiation to the chest area. Even though the implants had not turned out as I had hoped, I was still happy that I had the chance to try them. Now it's just me, and it is still by my choice, which makes all the difference in the world.

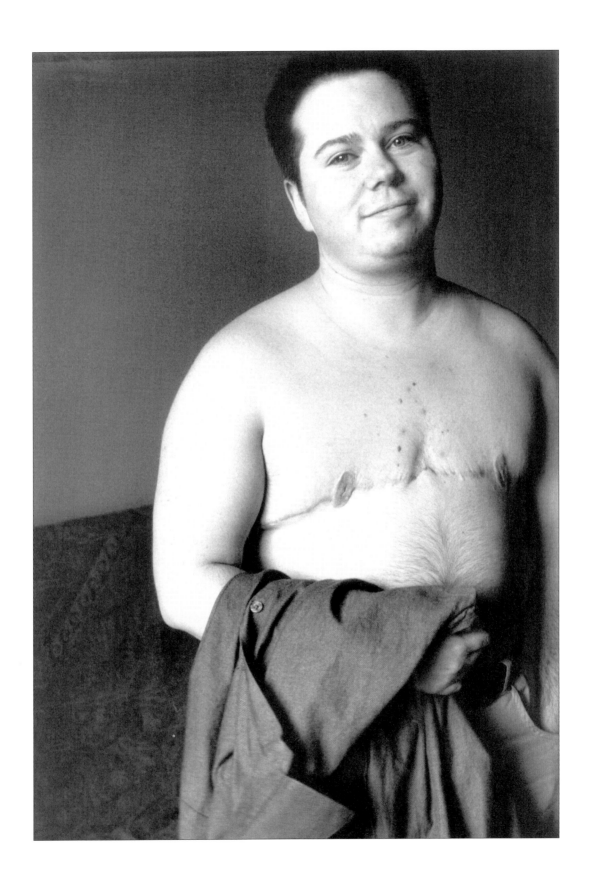

KYLE SCANLON
A Medical Necessity, A Life Necessity

In his transition from female to male, Kyle Scanlon initially had a breast reduction. A second surgery, gynaecomastia reduction, was performed five years later to completely remove the breasts and sculpt his chest. For Kyle, this procedure was "a medical necessity." Kyle speaks of the marked difference in response he received to the two surgeries and of the many other difficulties faced by someone transitioning.

Kyle was recently the Executive Director of the Lesbian, Gay, Bisexual YouthLine, and currently oversees the Meal Trans program at the 519 Church Street Community Centre. He has been a transsexual rights activist for many years and has been involved in a variety of projects profiling the experiences of transitioning. Kyle begins with excerpts from his journal from the time of his second surgery, and then continues with the story behind the surgeries.

Saturday, July 15, 2000

Officially now, instead of saying, "Less than two weeks till top surgery," I can say, "Just over one week till top surgery." It's hard to imagine that in the extremely near future, I will no longer have those breasts. I will no longer have to trouble myself with a binder. I'll be able to wear one shirt instead of dealing with the four-tiered system of putting on a sports bra, a binder, a t-shirt, and an outer shirt that I undergo currently. Being able to see the masculine contours of my chest underneath one shirt will go a long way towards helping me feel that my transition is more complete. By next summer, my scarring will be almost completely healed; if my past healing abilities are any indication, they will heal quite well. It'll be nice to take my shirt off in public eventually. If necrosis happens, and I resign myself to that as a possibility, I'll get a cosmetic tattoo. The main thing, as far as I'm concerned, is that I have proper contouring so that I can wear a t-shirt and look normal.

God, I can't believe it's going to happen. In a matter of weeks I'll no longer even have the post-surgical bandages to contend with. I'll be putting a shirt on over top of nothing — no bra, no binder, no extra t-shirt — and walking outside. I'll be wrapping a towel around my waist instead of my chest when I exit my morning shower. I'll be able to hug people without them feeling those breasts or binders. I'll no longer be a girl faking it, but a guy legit. It's funny how you don't realize you feel a certain way until the feeling is sitting right there in your gut. Right now I still feel like a fraud. I may be Kyle on my birth certificate, and my face is becoming more Kylesque every day, but every night when I go to bed and every morning when I wake up I still have this decidedly female body. Sure I have broader shoulders and hairier legs, arms and face, but what I've never been able to escape or overlook are those breasts. When I catch a glimpse of myself in the mirror, I still see those fucking tits and it undoes the process of establishing my new identity.

I'm glad this surgery is about to happen. I need it so badly for my sense of personhood to settle.

Tuesday, July 25, 2000

I'm boobless. It's 11:00 p.m. and I'm feeling great. If today is any indication of how the rest of my recovery will be, doubtless things shall go speedily. I was released from the clinic at 2:00 p.m., and have been awake and relatively active ever since. Certainly I've been mentally acute. My friend Carol called in the afternoon and asked, "Did you actually have the surgery?" She said my voice sounded so strong, it was hard to imagine I had been under the surgeon's knife just six hours earlier. Oddly, I don't feel that there's much to write tonight. Suffice it to say, I'm thrilled. On cloud nine. Happiness incarnate.

Thursday, July 27, 2000

I know I've been exceptionally silent in terms of writing about my surgery thus far, but I think my silence is because it's been so hard to know how to encapsulate the infinite number of thoughts and feelings I'm processing into just a few paragraphs. Perhaps I'll need to sound oafish, blunt, and shallow for now. For instance, my shirt hangs so beautifully. Can my first major expression about my surgery really be that my shirt hangs well? How puerile. But no, I guess it's not actually a statement about the shirt itself; it's about how I see myself. It's about seeing pieces of myself that I've never gotten to see before, but that I knew were there. That wonderful chest that was trapped underneath those damnable breasts is now visible. Notice how I never say "my breasts"; it's always "those breasts, those things that have nothing to do with me, those things that have absolutely nothing to do with any second of my future." Today I got a glimpse of my naked chest, of how it looks immediately post-surgery.

It looks like crap. But it also looks like it will look pretty good once it's healed. The scar line is fairly straight. The scars themselves are thin and the contours are good. My chest looks quite male. Well, it sure as hell doesn't look female anymore. Once I start working out, those chest muscles will look even better. My doctor has given me a chest that I will very easily be able to sculpt into a great set of pecs. I can't see my nipples yet. They're still hidden beneath the gauze layering that the surgeon sewed over the grafts, but they're beautifully small and they're in the right place, and that's really all I could hope for.

Thursday, August 3, 2000

I got to see my nipples for the first time today. The right one looks good, but it still has some healing to do and is struggling for survival. The left one, on the other hand, has a hole in it. *There's a hole in my nipple, dear Liza, dear Liza, there's a hole in my nipple, dear Liza, a hole.* My surgeon thinks the hole is likely a result of the infection; even though we caught it fairly quickly, it must have had enough time to destabilize the tissue underneath the nipple grafts. The good news: so I've got a small, pencil-width-sized hole in my left nipple that scar tissue can rebuild. And what would the colour of scar tissue be? Light pinky-red, very similar to the colour of the nipple itself. In the worst-case scenario, I'll have to get the tissue tattooed the right colour. It's not as if I'll be a nipple-hole freak for the rest of my life, after all. I'm okay with this. This was a risk I was comfortable taking. What's most important now is that my health is good, that I keep the incision line clean, that I keep taking care not to lift anything heavy, that I protect and foster my body's healing processes by taking vitamins, and that I get lots of rest.

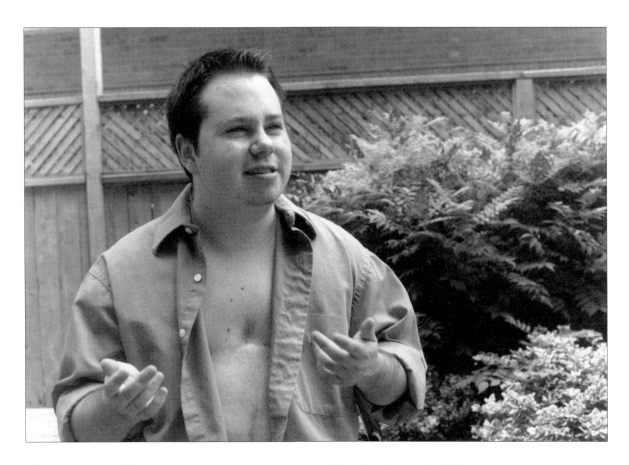

Saturday, August 5, 2000

I've been rubbing my chest with vitamin E. It's my way of attempting to keep the scarring to a minimum. The incision lines are so radically different from the ones from my previous surgery. With the reduction surgery, I think the weight of the remaining breast tissue pushed down on the stitching and must have caused the scars to stretch. But these lines are almost razor thin. Once they have some resolution and begin to fade, I can't imagine they'll be overly visible, especially not beneath the bountiful chest hair I expect I'll eventually have.

Tuesday, August 8, 2000

I've recently been pondering "passing," and have noticed that I've been *ma'amed* a lot since the surgery. The explanation one of my friends came up with makes some sense. I've just had surgery, so I'm likely feeling vulnerable, and vulnerability, or the expression of it, is often associated with femininity and femaleness. Three different friends have also told me that since my surgery, I'm moving and walking differently and giving off a different energy than I did before. That's probably true, and as odd as this may sound, I think part of it is because I'm not binding. The process of binding my breasts was a part of my getting-in-touch-with-my-masculinity exercise. Now that I'm no longer doing it, I feel slightly unsettled. After all, that binding literally provided a thick layer of protection between me and the outside world. Now I'm trying to get used to being me without my armour. Never in my adult life have I ever ventured outside so unprotected, so bare. I'm scared of being seen so clearly, but I'll cope.

Thursday, August 31, 2000

Good news. The surgeon and I will be meeting for a small revisionary session in late September to clean up the scars even more. And something occurred while I was in his office today. I noticed that taking off my shirt in his presence was a completely different experience for me than it was the first time I had been in there with him. The first time, when he wanted to see what kind of canvas he had to work with, I craned my neck up and away, embarrassed. I needed to hide the sight of those breasts even from myself. That first time, I felt grossly on display, extremely vulnerable. Today, taking off my shirt was a piece of cake. I was just a guy taking off my shirt. I was a guy before, too, but I was a guy who had the misfortune of having breasts. No wonder I felt embarrassed.

I had a difficult time deciding whether or not I could be a part of a project entitled "My Breasts, My Choice." As a transsexual man, the whole idea of having breasts was absolutely painful for me; hence, I had the surgery to remove those breasts. The name of the project itself was like having my status as a female reasserted. I wasn't comfortable with that. What made it easier to choose to be involved was that it was open to biological men talking about their various chest surgeries as well. Clearly this book isn't only about women's breast surgeries.

Another part of my decision to be involved was so that I could educate. I'm a female-to-male transsexual (FTM). Mentally and psychologically, I now see myself as a guy, but the body I was born with was clearly female. When the doctors saw my body at birth, they assigned a female gender to me and my parents gave me a female name. I was raised as a girl. At puberty, my body went through the same growth spurt that all female bodies go through and I developed breasts. After I ultimately came out as a transsexual man, I was in a position of being a guy who had breasts.

In 1995, I had a breast reduction in the hopes that it would allow me to feel more at peace with myself, but that wasn't enough. I soon understood that my issue with my breasts wasn't with their size, but with having them period. I realized I needed to make a transition from female to male. In order to strengthen my sense of self-identity as a transsexual man and to have a more masculine, male-contoured body I needed to have those breasts removed. I started taking male hormones, but I couldn't pass very well as a man when I had breasts! I began walking around in the world using a male name. People were using male pronouns for me, and I was growing facial hair. But when I went home at night, I would unwrap this rigmarole of bandages I used to bind my breasts down to hide them from people. I still had to deal with my breasts. So I decided to have the surgery as soon as I was able to afford it. In fact, I went into debt to have this surgery.

The surgery wasn't cosmetic for me in any sense; rather it was a medical necessity, a life necessity. Having the surgery was as necessary as having oxygen to breathe. A lot of FTM men, including myself, don't even think of breast surgery as breast reduction or breast removal; we think of it as treating our gynaecomastia. *Gynaecomastia* is the medical term used to describe a male with female-like or excess breast tissue. Many men with this condition choose surgery to remove that excess breast tissue. When I filled out my forms with the surgeon, he asked, "What are you here for?" I wrote *gynaecomastia*. Internally, my vision of myself was that I was a guy who had excess breast tissue that had to go.

FIRST SURGERY:
Reduction

In 1995, I identified as a lesbian. I was in a semi-permanent relationship that I thought would last for quite a while. My partner and I were living together. I was a 36DD, and on the surface, my concern with my breasts at that point was back problems. Because of their size, I couldn't jog or exercise. It was too painful. But underneath that, I also knew I hated those breasts as they were. I didn't quite understand why. I only knew that I felt they didn't fit my body. I thought, Maybe a breast reduction would help, for physical and mental reasons.

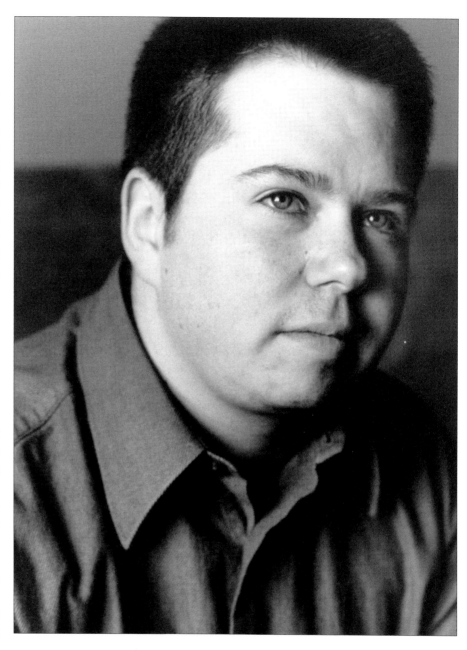

My partner was pretty open to this idea. Admittedly, I was a little concerned. What if something went wrong? What if I lost all sensation? But the truth was, the more I thought about it the more I knew I just really wanted it done. When the surgeon asked me, "How big do you want your breasts to be in the end?" I said, "Very, very small."

When I woke up after the surgery, my breasts weren't nearly as small as I thought they were going to be, or as I had wanted them to be, and this was very painful. I felt that I had gone through the whole surgical process for nothing. I didn't fully understand then that what I'd wanted were no breasts at all. Part of me must have known, but not all of me, not fully consciously. At that point, I didn't recognize I was FTM; I thought I was a dyke with gender issues.

My breasts had been so large. It seems strange to talk about their size; it's hard for me to talk about "my breasts" at all. In my mind, they weren't even supposed to *be*. They were like an invading enemy lodged in my body. I didn't talk about them and I didn't want them to be a part of me. I just didn't like them, but there they were and I had to cope with them.

One of the things that used to totally incense me was the way some men would look at me — they'd look at my chest. I lived most of my life with my arms crossed in front of my chest because I hated that part of my body so much. I have nothing against breasts on women, but I am not a woman. I didn't have the words for it at the time.

I definitely didn't get what I wanted from the first surgery. What I'd wanted were "very, very small" breasts. Instead I went from having very large to medium large breasts. The change was noticeable, but it wasn't nearly the change I wanted. When I reminded the surgeon later that I'd wanted to be "very, very small," she said, "All women say that, but it's not really what they want." I felt raped, assaulted — medically assaulted — by someone deciding she knew better than I did what I wanted. Her comments and her making that surgical decision infuriated me. Now I tell anyone who will listen, "Do not leave anything to chance." When it comes to having any cosmetic medical or surgical procedure, tell the surgeon *exactly* what you want. Use drawings or pictures to give the surgeon an idea of what you're looking for. Be really clear and go to extreme lengths to communicate your ideas to the surgeon because the rest of your life is going to be riding on having been as precise as possible about what you want.

The surgeon left me with some big scars, but I'd anticipated that. I lost most of the sensation in my nipples, but I'd been prepared for that too. In fact, the results of my surgery deepened my sense that those breasts weren't mine. I still had these globs of flesh that had no purpose at all. This was an interesting time in my life as I tried to figure out my feelings. Was I happy that I'd had the surgery? Was I upset that I'd had the surgery? Was I more disappointed than pleased? For a long time I wasn't really sure how I felt.

Fortunately, I had some support. Many people around me assured me that they understood what I was going through. They told me they understood that my breasts were large and that their size just wasn't appropriate on a very small person. I didn't face any dissent for having had that surgery. In fact, my parents drove me home from the hospital and helped care for me. All my female friends were very supportive.

SECOND SURGERY:
Gynaecomastia

For the second surgery, however, the reactions I received were completely different. Everybody freaked out. "You're having your breasts removed? Oh, my god! This is mutilation!" They had been able to understand the reasoning behind that first surgery and wanting to be more traditionally attractive, wanting to have breasts that were more size-appropriate for my body. But the second surgery, which I saw as being equivalent to life-sustaining oxygen, they all saw as mutilation. They asked, "Why would you want to do this to yourself?"

I found this response really interesting. Culturally, we have a standard of what a beautiful woman is

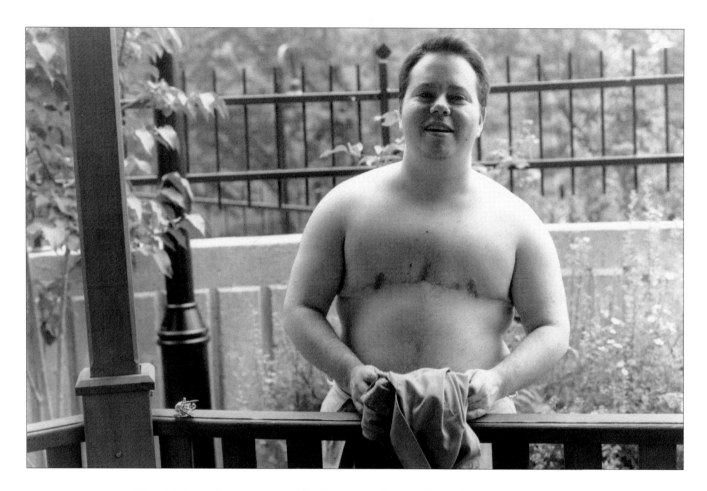

supposed to look like. With the first surgery, I felt like people were saying, "Oh, of course, you want to mould yourself into that more perfect vision of female beauty. That's completely understandable. Go ahead. Go under the knife, put yourself under anaesthetic, have someone do horrible things to you while you're fast asleep. That's okay." They approved of my decision. But having the second surgery to correct the gynaecomastia, which for me was purely for survival, people saw as a decision to mutilate myself. I saw their reaction as trans-phobia. Fortunately, in terms of support for the second surgery, I already knew a lot of trans-identified people, both men and women, who understood that I had a mental and psychological need to have the gynaecomastia corrected, a need that had

nothing to do with aesthetics.

By the time I was ready to have my second surgery, I found myself, along with other people in the transgender community in Toronto, scrambling to find a doctor willing to perform surgery without psychiatric letters of referral. For cosmetic surgery, people don't need a letter from a psychiatrist. But to perform a "transsexual" surgery, the standard guidelines regarding the treatment of transsexuals recommend we get letters from referring psychiatrists stating that this person "has been found to be of sound mind and is able to make an informed, consenting decision to have transsexual surgery, is experiencing gender dysphoria, and has been diagnosed with gender identity disorder." Then the doctor can go ahead and cut the person open. And so the hunt was on to find a doctor in Toronto who wouldn't require letters. I probably could have gotten those letters eventually — after years of therapy and monitoring by a gender clinic — but that wouldn't have helped me in my immediate situation. I was dealing with binding down my medium-sized breasts to make them invisible. This was mentally and physically painful, to say the least.

Finally, another FTM man I knew found a surgeon willing to perform chest surgery without reference letters. Word got out about this surgeon, and the next thing you knew, about ten of us had either already seen him or were scheduled to see him! He had only performed surgery for one FTM before, however, so we had to train him and his staff in transgender issues, in things like using the right pronouns despite what it said on our health cards. This surgery experience really contrasted with my first one. I didn't have to train my first surgeon; she knew she was doing a breast reduction and treated it simply as that. It was a standard procedure for her and before the surgery she'd come in, drawn her little diagram, and then left. We didn't actually discuss anything. My second surgeon and his staff, however, were very open to learning. If they couldn't remember, they would ask, "What pronoun am I supposed to use?" until they got it. We participated in a bit more give-and-take this time around, which was important.

I needed them to know that they were operating on a man. Regardless of the fact that they were operating on breasts and on a person whose health card said "female," they were operating on a man. I needed to make sure that even when I was asleep, they were calling me "he" and using my male name. I needed to make sure that even the anaesthetist knew that I was a guy. If I could feel sure about these things, then I knew I would feel protected even when I wasn't able to be awake to protect myself. These concerns aren't the ones that people normally think about when they go for surgery.

Another FTM guy I once knew said that what was really important for him was that his breasts be cut off not in hate, but in love. He wanted to feel that the surgeon was sculpting his chest, not simply removing his breasts. I sort of felt the same way. I wanted this to be about my chest, not about my breasts, about moving toward rather than moving away, about becoming rather than about losing. I wanted this surgery to be a celebration of self!

After I had the surgery, I sped through the healing process. This was a very exhilarating time. I would say, "Anybody want to see my scars, my chest?" There was something so thrilling about having a male chest. It didn't and doesn't look perfect, but it's mine. And it's much, much closer to the way I want it to be. There's something so wonderfully simple about walking out of a shower and wrapping a towel around my waist, like men do, instead of around my chest, like women do. Those are little things, but they're important.

I finally felt some persistence and congruence between who I felt myself to be and how I looked that had been missing before. It was the best thing in the world. I took a walk in a park north of the city with a friend about six weeks after my gynaecomastia surgery. He took his shirt off and then I did, too. That day was the first time I had ever taken my shirt off in public. I was outside, a part of nature — the sky, the sun, the trees and me. It was exhilarating. Other guys could take that for granted. Not me.

I am very happy with my new chest; however, I had done a lot of research before I started. Based on my experience, I want to encourage people to be as fully aware as possible of what to expect from a cosmetic surgery before having any procedures done. Being aware of the risks and asking, "Could I live with the worst-case scenario if it happened?" is important. One

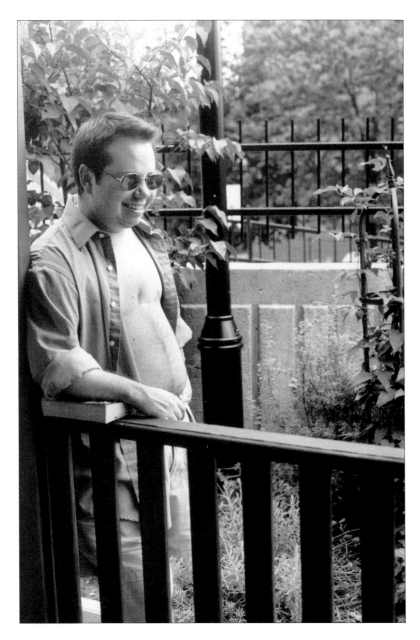

more likely that it would eventually fill in, but I had no idea what it would ultimately look like. Before having the surgery, I knew that a hole was possible if I got an infection. I had to ask myself, "Is this an acceptable risk?" And I realized it was.

In the weeks before I went into surgery, I wrote pages and pages in my journal questioning myself about different scenarios. I wrote: "If this happens, will I accept it? Will I be able to cope with *that* outcome?" As long as I kept coming up with "yes," then I knew I was okay. If there had been one time when I came up with "no," then I would have had to re-evaluate. The cost-to-benefit ratio was really clear: I had a goal and my goal was to look good in a shirt. For me it wasn't so much about what I looked like with my clothes off, but about how I would look with a shirt on. Knowing the latter was my goal meant that, even if things went wrong — bad scars or destabilized skin tissue — none of that would change the fact that, in a shirt, I would look much more like a guy. Once I knew I felt clear on that, I could proceed.

Now that I have had the surgery, I can talk about it. My scars are prominent. I apply vitamin E, zinc, MSM (methyl sulphonyl methane, an organic sulphur compound for repairing body tissue), and vitamin K to help reduce them. They're fading, so these things seem to be working. I look at treating my scars not only as a form of self-care, but also self-love. Whenever I'm putting these lotions on, I feel that I am

of the things that happened with my gynaecomastia surgery was that I got an infection. As a result, some of the tissue around one of my nipples became destabilized and caved in. I then had to deal with the fact that I might always have extended scar tissue there. It was reclaiming my ability to touch myself with love and acceptance, which is something I hadn't done for a very long time.

I no longer have any sensation in my nipples, but to me, that's a fair trade. In a way, I have more sensation now in my chest overall than I ever had before because I'm more willing to allow people to touch me there. This change in my willingness makes all the difference in the world.

When I initially began identifying as a guy, I stopped wanting to be sexual at all. I felt as if I only had two negative options in terms of sexual contact: I could either try to pretend that I didn't have breasts, which was ridiculous and impossible to do, or I could choose abstinence. After the surgery, I felt much more comfortable. I felt more options were open to me and I started thinking about my sexuality and sensuality again. I am ready to have a positive relationship with my body now, something I haven't had in a very, very long time.

During the course of this experience, I have become more aware of the difference between gender cues and sex cues. Most people probably don't think much about this difference. People in the queer community, though, think about it all the time. For example, when people in straight society identify dykes or lesbians as men, straight society is looking at their gender cues — short hair and boy's clothes. They're not looking at the physical features that define a person as being female — smaller jaw-line, smaller shoulders, wider hips. Ironically, when I'm in a straight community, I pass very well as a man because I have all the right gender cues. Some of my sex cues are also more male now that I've been on testosterone for a year. My jaw-line is wider, my shoulders are wider, and my hips are smaller. But in the queer community, where people tend to look past gender cues to sex cues, they often read FTMs early in transition as lesbians. This is very frustrating. In the very place that is supposed to be our home, our safe haven, I feel the least safe. No one ever gets the pronouns right. Sometimes I actually feel more comfortable in the straight community. I never would have thought that could be the case.

I would really like people to stop labelling others quite so much, and rather allow people to label themselves or not to label themselves as they see fit. For instance, I'm a man unlike other men. I'm a man who wants to be welcome in lesbian spaces. I'm a man who used to be a dyke, who is now bisexual and dates gay men. What label is there to accommodate all that?

I've become aware that gender and sexual orientation are absolutely unrelated concepts. Obviously something has changed if I say that I was a dyke and now I'm bisexual, but I'm not talking about my sexual orientation. I'm talking about my understanding of my own body, and my ability to deal with my body. When I had a body that was much more overtly female, during the few times that I was with men intimately it was very obvious that I was with "men being with a woman." I couldn't handle that. When I was a woman with women, suddenly all the roles about what men were supposed to do with women were tossed out the window. We were just two people fucking, and that was okay. I wanted freedom from those roles. I could have that freedom with women, but I didn't feel I could have it with men, which was frustrating, because I wanted it with men too.

Now that I feel free from the gender-role stereotypes, I date men without that baggage. I have shifted. I'm more comfortable with my body now. I have always been attracted to men; but as I was, I just felt I couldn't be with them. Now I'm able to be more honest about who I'm attracted to, and more able to act on it.

Not that there still aren't issues for me to deal with, however. People are always wondering, "Who exactly would want you? You're a man without a dick." It comes up a lot — "Who would ever want *that?*" The truth is, I don't know. I don't have an answer. I don't know if many people will, and I have to live with that. If my choices are either to be a person who can't stand his own body but is deemed attractive to others, or to be a person who's much happier with who he is and has to be patient in finding a partner who's truly attracted to him as he is, then it's not a hard choice. I'd rather be happy with myself. Besides, if truth be told, there is no way a person is going to be attractive to others unless that person believes him or herself to be worthy of attraction.

I think I now have a much better chance of attracting the kind of person who will be attracted to me, because I'm out there. I'm an activist. I'm more self-confident. I feel more comfortable with my body. It may take a while for all the pieces of my puzzle to fit into place, but I'm confident that they will, in time.

I like to remember something that happened fairly recently. I went to see an old friend and her mom. When her mom was saying good-bye, she did that thing that women often do with men: she put her hand on my chest and said, "It was nice to see you." Her hand just rested there. It felt more genuine than anything I'd ever experienced. No one would have made that gesture so casually before. No straight woman, especially not Kathy's mom, would have ever put her hand where my breasts used to be. That she did it so casually felt as if she had accepted the fact that I was a guy. Her touch on my chest felt fundamentally different. It was powerful, rewarding, sensual, comforting and ultimately affirming.

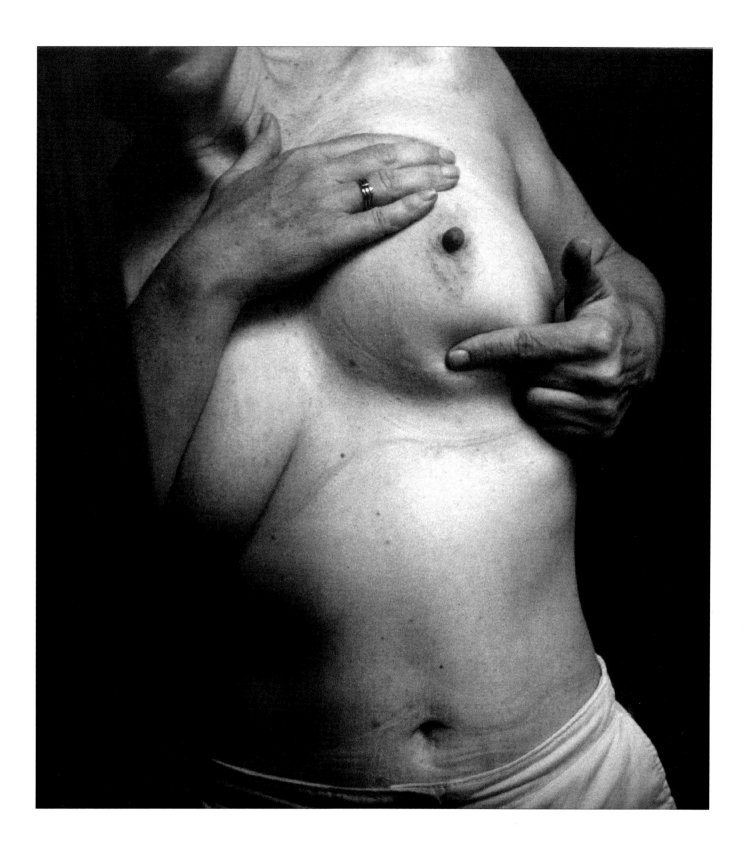

ANGELA'S STORY
Into the Light

Angela has had two primary scares of breast cancer. She has undergone mammography, biopsy, coring (breast calcification sampling) and lumpectomy. The growths have all been benign. Participating in both the photo exhibit of My Breasts, My Choice *and in the book has been a process of "bringing my breasts into the light" — a part of Angela's emotional and spiritual healing journey. Angela is the mother to two adopted sons and sister to Laura, who is also part of* My Breasts, My Choice. *Angela has chosen to maintain partial anonymity in the project.*

For health reasons, it has been important for me to reclaim my breasts, to know I have the right to enjoy them, to feel them.

I'm fifty and I have had breast surgery twice, a lumpectomy in 1994 and breast calcification sampling in 1997. My breast tissue is dense. I've never breast-fed, and I've never given birth. Research has found that these factors increase my risk for breast cancer.

My breasts are active, with changes in the tissue occurring quite regularly. These changes are all concerns for me and I don't think the changes are a good sign. My mother's sister lost both breasts and eventually died from breast cancer. When I was eleven years old, I cut myself off from my breasts because of the way my family treated breasts and me once I had them. This was a young age and I think I have a lot of energy locked in my breasts.

I am the oldest daughter of five children. I was the first to develop breasts and discover what that meant in our family. One day, my mother and I were in my bedroom and I was complaining about my chest being sore. My mother said, "You're blossoming." I was eleven, just hitting puberty, and very innocent. In my innocence, I went downstairs where my father and brothers were watching TV. I stood in front of them, pulled up my t-shirt, and said, "I'm blossoming." I knew right away that I had done a "dirty" thing. That was the beginning of having breasts.

In my family there was a lot of shame around breasts and bodies and being female. There was a lot of attention placed on modesty and on not doing what girls normally do at that age. Makeup and pantyhose were not allowed. As we got older, my sisters and I learned to wear heavy clothing, and tried desperately to hide our bodies. I dressed in the closet. Whole years went by when I didn't see my own breasts. Somehow, like a nun, I was even able to bathe without seeing them.

My father used to say, "Put your housecoat on around your brothers." In my father's household, it seemed like an outrage to grow breasts. And at the same time, my home also had a highly sexually charged atmosphere. When my oldest brother was twelve, he showed obvious, public signs of acting out sexually and was always very crude. For many years, he and my father were guilty of incest with me and my sisters, Christine and Laura.

About the time I reached the end of elementary school, my father went bankrupt. We went from having a lot of money to having no money, and had to sell our house and rent a much smaller one. My sisters and I shared one room. It was into this room that my brother John would come at night. Sometimes I'd wake up and he'd be standing at the end of the bed, staring at me. Other times I woke up to find him in my bed, touching my breasts.

During that time I gained a lot of weight. I think I was to trying to shield myself from John, because the weight disappeared as soon as he left for university. I didn't go on a diet or exercise. The minute he left home, I dropped some of my need for bulk and protection. Some years later, my sister Christine reminded me of another experience concerning my breasts. When my brother John left home, I started dating. When I finally allowed a boy to "feel me up," Christine had asked, "How was it?" I had thought it would be great, but it wasn't. I didn't understand why my neck and ears had more feeling than my breasts. All I said to Christine was, "It was really quite a lemon. I couldn't feel a thing." Christine was the first one to question why I couldn't feel anything.

My relationship with my sister Christine has been an intense and difficult one. When we were young, Christine was beautiful. I was treated as the plain one, and was often compared to my namesake aunt. People always talked about what beautiful hands Aunt Angela had, but basically she was the one to do the housework. She was also very heavy. The message was that Christine was beautiful, Laura was pretty, and Angela had nice hands like her Aunt Angela. One day I looked at my aunt and realized that she was actually quite beautiful. She also led a very interesting life, but it took a while for me to figure that out.

We all had roles in the family and my role was to take care of everyone. When Christine was born, she felt almost like *my* child. I remember thinking, "Now we're even. We've got two boys and two girls." I could never understand why she didn't want to align herself with me. I had thought we would unite and fight the battle of the sexes! Instead, we battled against each other. Christine was bright, witty, bitchy, dramatic, and tough to get along with. In fact our relationship was very difficult emotionally. She had a lot of anger toward me because I was so compliant and was always trying to keep the peace at home. I was afraid of my father's rage. The nicer I acted, the more angry Christine became with me for trying to maintain the status quo. I didn't catch on then why I couldn't get along with my sister. The more I tried, the worse it got. About the time I left home, however, Christine noticed a shift in my attitude. She said that when I lost weight, *I* became bitchy. It was true; I didn't behave like the servant anymore. I was more into my own life and quite proud of it.

After leaving my family home, I became sexually active. I went on the pill, lost more weight and my breasts became smaller. I was happy to have smaller breasts. Oddly, at the same time, Christine grew very large breasts after having been small-breasted. I think this change was hard for her, given that it seemed to happen very suddenly; it was almost like an after-effect of my leaving. She was now the oldest daughter at home.

Then, when I was twenty-four, Christine called me on her twenty-first birthday from a psychiatric ward, declaring that my father had been admitted to the hospital and was about to die. I didn't know why Christine was in a psychiatric ward or why my father was in a hospital. The physicians didn't tell us that my father might die, or how serious his illness was, but Christine had been right. Within ten days, my father was dead. That was Christine's first visit to the psychiatric ward.

Over the years, Christine battled schizophrenia and was in and out of the psychiatric wards. Amazingly, during this time she also completed her law degree with honours. Christine always decided when she needed to go back to the hospital. Not until the summer she was twenty-six, when she had a severe psychotic breakdown, did a friend commit her. After that experience, Christine said that she would never ever go into a psychiatric ward again.

A social worker at the hospital had told us that Christine had a fifty-fifty chance of committing suicide before the age of fifty. She said we had to start thinking about how we would take care of ourselves if this happened. This was the first time I really understood that she was sick, and it made me pay attention.

During the following year our relationship was quite peaceful, because I was more open to her. In a situation like that, you're supposed to ask the person, "Are you planning on committing suicide?" When I asked her this in June, Christine answered, "I've never been farther from it."

In August, when she was twenty-seven years old, Christine committed suicide. This year is the twentieth anniversary of her death.

I found healing around my sister Christine difficult initially. There is always a certain amount of guilt around a suicide and I feel I let her down. Before she took her life, Christine talked about the incest with my brother, but I wasn't open to hearing it. My response to her was that whatever had happened was no big deal. "We lived in an alcoholic, violent family. There was sexual abuse, and I survived it. I'm going to get on with my life. I'm not going to dwell on it." Essentially I was saying that I was not interested in hearing about her experience because it was too painful. It was dev-

astating to have her commit suicide after I had not been supportive of her talking about the incest.

Apparently Christine laid out a funeral dress before she died. I never saw it — the police certainly weren't going to worry about whether she was in the right dress. I don't know what happened to the dress. To clothe her in the casket, I gave the funeral home some of my clothes, including my bra and my favourite red shirt. It felt very intimate to give her my clothes.

After her death, I went into chronic grieving. Eventually I started therapy, which allowed me to deal with my family history, Christine's death, the incest and my body. Through therapy, massage and dreams, Christine became more present to me. We are close now, close in a way that life did not permit.

About five years after Christine died, I had a breakdown. I fell apart and could no longer function at work. I took time off, and near the end of that time, I had a dream about Christine. In the dream she came to me, and I said to her, "I want to go with you." My longing to leave with her was huge. She said, "It'll be soon enough." I remember what she was wearing, where she was, how her hair looked, though I saw just a glimpse of her: Her face was veiled by her thick, black hair, and she was wearing a red floral-pattern dress. (I have since wondered if it was the dress she had laid out for her funeral.)

In the second part of the dream, I said to her, "While you have a direct link to God, could you get me a baby?" It was less than half a year after that dream that my first son came along. I believe that Christine made our first adoption happen, because we hadn't even been on a list for adopting a child. After not being able to get pregnant, we hadn't pursued adoption at all — the possibility for disappointment was too big. Somehow, though, through people we didn't even know, the birth mother of our two sons came into our life.

Six years later, I found the dream written down. I reread it, surprised, because I hadn't remembered the second part. A few days after that, we got the call about our second son. Part of my healing has definitely come from becoming a mother. My husband and I now have two wonderful kids through adoption, and their coming into our lives is, for me, connected with Christine.

When I was a teenager, my father used to stare at my breasts. He stared with rage, but also with sexual energy. I was always trying to make myself more and more invisible. When I began therapy, I focused mainly on my father. For me, whatever had happened with my father was worse than anything else.

Before my first son was born, I had a series of bear dreams which helped me to come to terms with my father's incest with me. The details of the bears were very clear, and the dreams were quite scary.

In my first dream, when I saw a grizzly bear, I knew I had to pretend to be dead; otherwise this bear would kill me. At some point I knew that I couldn't play dead anymore, so I slid down the mountain as fast as I could. I ended up in a very small cell with bars around me. I was with Canada's most-wanted criminal, and the front of his trousers was right up against my face. I woke up calling my brother John's name. In the beginning of the dream, I had been calling my father's name, but somehow it became John's. The two of them were somehow linked.

My father was a big man. He would actually scratch his back against the doorjamb. He used to play "bear" with us when we were kids. We had to hop on the couch or the "bear" would get us. He had bear energy.

In another bear dream I was in a cottage. A black bear was trying to break in through an open window when a giant cowboy rode along on a horse. He chased after the bear. I didn't feel any fear, but thought, You don't have to chase the bear; the bear has wandered off. Somehow there came to be a healing energy in the bear. I began to reclaim that wild part of myself.

In one of my last bear dreams, there was a beautiful image of two polar bears floating by on an ice floe. The image of the bears in the dream was enclosed in a circle. When I woke up, I painted the image. I looked at the polar bears and didn't feel any terror. Instead, I felt a lot of mutual respect. A shift had occurred in what the bears represented: they went from attacking bears to respecting bears. This shift came from realizing that something horrible had happened with my father and I didn't have to contain it anymore.

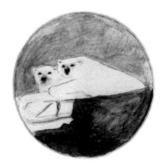

Healing around my brother John began just prior to my second son's birth. I was doing a type of body healing work called "Tibetan pulsing." In one session, the woman I was working with asked, "Can you feel the chill in the room?" I wasn't 100 percent sure, but it was obviously very real to her. She said, "It's your sister," meaning Christine. "She is quite demanding." It was odd because I hadn't talked much with this woman about what Christine was like. The body worker said, "Christine's quite witty, but in-my-face. She's angry because she was the one who was hurt so much, and you weren't. She doesn't see that you were hurt by your brother's incest." The body worker invited Christine to feel what had really happened, to witness my pain as well. Christine's response was that I had to heal my breasts.

After the session was over, I asked the body worker what Christine looked like. She described Christine exactly as I had seen her in my first dream, with her thick dark hair and the red floral dress. That experience prompted me to ask myself seriously, What does it mean to heal my breasts? How do I take care of my breasts? I

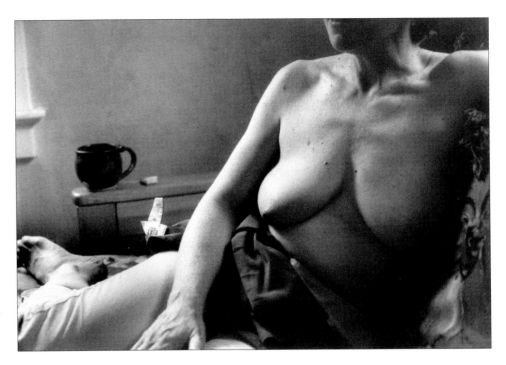

had already done a lot of work around my father in my therapy, and yet there was obviously something I still had to do.

My brother John has lived in another province for over twenty-five years. In 1985 he was diagnosed with a psychiatric disorder. For the longest time there was no contact between us, and then, about six years ago, he started calling me once a week. One day he called and apologized about the incest, even though I had never talked about it with him. He said, "I know that I may have done degrading things to you, and I want to say it's entirely my fault. I'm sorry." I said, "I hear what you're saying." But I couldn't say, "I forgive you."

It seemed like an act of grace for him to apologize, even though it wasn't a full disclosure. So, through the phone calls, I allowed him more into my life, but I thought to myself, The next time I see you will be when I go to your funeral. It seemed like a fair thing.

And then, two summers ago, John ended up in my

city and at my door. My older brother had told him that John could no longer live with him. When I opened the door, I saw that John looked just like my father. I wouldn't have recognized him as John, except that he had his voice.

I let him stay, but I slept in one son's room and my husband slept in the other son's room the whole time he was there. John slept in the basement. For me, there were two energies to his stay. Part of me was happy to have him there, but with his overweight body, white hair and undershirts, another part of me felt like he was a white slug in the basement.

At one point during his stay, John started talking about what a great body I had in high school. My husband said to me, "You should tell him not to talk like this in front of your eight year old son." I said, "Why don't you say something to him?" because it was really hard for me to say anything. Even twenty-five years later, John was still sexually charged around me.

I got through the insanity of his stay and never confronted him, which is odd, because I can be quite direct. I just wanted him out of my house.

Once home, he began writing letters that ended with, "I'm sending this by Angela-mail — snail mail with breasts." He was creating this image of me as a snail dragging her breasts through the mud.

Not long afterwards, I had a final dream with Christine in it in which she said, "I told you to heal your breasts." In the dream, I saw an image of bringing my breasts into the light. After this, I was able to confront John for the first time. I asked him directly not to use "snail mail" anymore and curtailed contact with him. Now I don't know if I'll even go to his funeral.

FIRST SURGERY:
Lumpectomy, Right Breast

I am not great at checking my breasts. My breasts are lumpy and the self-exam has never felt satisfactory. I often find lumps that I rationalize away. However, in 1994 I found a lump on the underside of my right breast that felt different — foreign and hard. My doctor assured me that since it was on the rim of the breast, that was an unlikely place for a malignant lump. Regardless, he made an appointment for me with an oncologist.

After the oncologist examined my breasts and reviewed mammograms, he told me that I had to have a needle biopsy. He explained that the pain of freezing the breast and the pain of the biopsy were equivalent. The needle biopsy was done immediately, before I had time to react. I was surprised that it was not very painful. It was unsuccessful, however, because the lump was solid and the doctor was unable to draw out a sample.

The oncologist told me that the lump was likely not cancerous, but the only way to know for sure was by doing a lumpectomy. The question was whether I could live with the uncertainty if I didn't have it. He noted that the lump was close to the surface, and therefore easily accessible. A lumpectomy could be done in day surgery, using a local anaesthetic. I immediately opted for the surgery.

My husband and young son accompanied me to the hospital. Because of the local anaesthetic, there was no pain. I did not like being conscious during the incision — I knew when the doctor was cutting into my breast. He told me that, on the basis of his visual inspection, the lump was likely benign, but this required confirmation through laboratory testing. I regret that I never looked at the lump myself; I imagine it as a slippery, greyish mass.

Following the surgery, I felt like a bird with a wounded wing — vulnerable and sad. In a dream, the lump became an acorn that I planted at the base of a tree, which seemed to symbolize both a death and a birth. I felt disconnected from my breast, betrayed by it, angry that I might be being penalized because I was infertile — I knew that not giving birth to a baby increased my risk of developing breast cancer. For a few weeks, I felt sore and tender. I had to avoid carrying heavy things, including my recently adopted child, which he did not understand. My friends were supportive, sharing their own experiences, which helped reduce my anxiety. My family was least able to offer support. I think the possibility of cancer was too frightening for them, particularly since my aunt had died of breast cancer at the age of fifty-one.

I experienced anxiousness marked by brief periods of sheer terror before the surgery and again following surgery as I waited for a diagnosis. My feelings

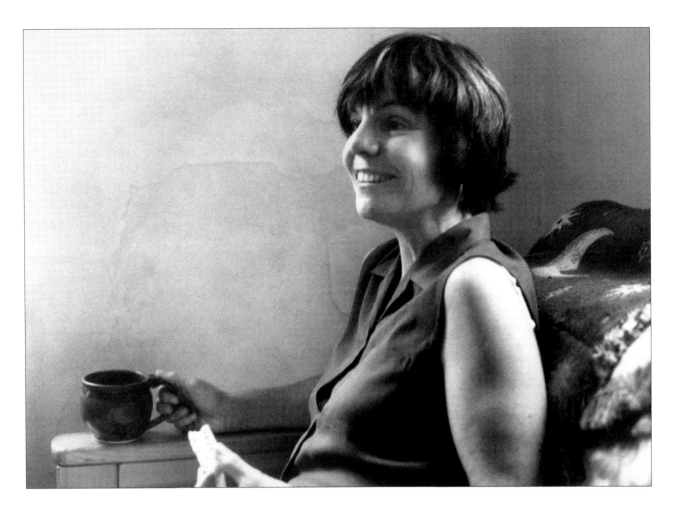

were tempered though by the thought that I was likely one of the lucky ones — that I was one of the nine out of ten who had lumps that were benign. I had difficulty allowing myself to have these feelings, given the likelihood of a non-cancerous result, and knowing that others would not be so lucky. Even though it was a short wait, the time felt surreal.

I received the diagnosis about two weeks after the surgery: benign, as anticipated. With the diagnosis, I felt a renewed sense of the preciousness of my life.

That same year, I developed severe skin rashes and the first of what has become essentially an annual bout of bronchitis. That trio of health issues awakened in me the need to try to understand what was going on in my body. I felt that my body was demanding my attention and that the price of not listening would become greater over time. I started having regular healing body-work sessions doing the Tibetan pulsing. Through the body-work, I came to the awareness that the activity in my right breast was linked to blocked memories and emotions from my family's past. I also joined a long-term study on the effects of a low-fat diet and possible reduction in rates of breast cancer. I continue to participate in the study and generally follow a low-fat diet.

Second Surgery:
Calcification Pattern, Left Breast

In 1997, my left breast developed irregularities. During my annual mammogram, the technician took extra time. Then, instead of being given the okay to go home, I was asked to have additional mammograms. Although I was wary at the time, I disregarded my unease until I received a phone call asking me to return for yet another mammogram of my left breast. I felt dread. I needed to talk about it immediately, and fortunately, a friend worked close by. She was the first of many that I told my fears to. I began to have an urge to tell my story, even to strangers. That night I had a dream that this time I was going to have the fight of my life.

At my follow-up appointment, everything felt ominous — the empty waiting room, the technician waiting to see me, the receptionist announcing that I had arrived. The hospital's newest mammogram machine was used, and the technician seemed to take special care in making the images. I did not have the heart to carry on my usual banter.

The next week I received a phone call asking me to return yet again to have another set of mammograms done. I called my doctor. She set up an oncology appointment for me, rather than have me go for a fourth round of mammograms. It was with the same oncologist as before.

The issue this time was a suspicious calcification pattern that could have been associated with cancer that was on my ribcage located deep under my left breast. Because it did not involve a lump, neither a needle biopsy nor lumpectomy would work. The oncologist proposed "coring," a process using wires placed in the breast and guided with the assistance of mammography. The procedure, which is not consid-ered surgery, would entail only a small incision. Multiple cores, or samples, of tissue could be taken from the same incision point, which meant faster recovery and less scarring. I found very little information in the literature about the links between calcification and breast cancer, which left me with many unanswered questions. This time I was really terrified. The possibility that I might have cancer felt more real than it had the first time. I pleaded with any and all higher powers to protect me.

My husband again accompanied me for the procedure. We waited more than two hours before discovering that my mammograms had been misplaced. I was reluctant to have another mammogram. As I was midway in my menstrual cycle, my breast was less full and it flattened too well on the mammogram plate. This was not a good thing. The doctor felt that the coring procedure under local anaesthetic would be unsafe because of the flattening of my breast; without more bulk in my breast, there was a risk the needle might come out the other side. Accordingly, surgery was recommended. They booked me for another day.

When the night before the surgery finally arrived, I had everything in place, including child care and a drive to the hospital. Although I kept reminding myself that I had enough time, I lay awake worrying about the need to shower and shave under my arms in the morning, and about making it downtown in time.

Preparation included the insertion of wires into my breast for guidance during the procedure. The process was long and involved and entailed remaining perfectly still, often for over half an hour at a time, in awkward and uncomfortable positions while attached to the mammogram machine. I had a strong urge to run away down the hospital hall, dragging the machine with me. Thankfully, the technician helped me calm down. I needed the wheelchair that was waiting for me following the procedure! I felt I had shown courage in making it through this.

I relaxed once the surgery preparation was completed. I joked with the nurses, and enjoyed and felt comforted by the camaraderie of the surgical team. I instinctively felt that they were high-energy and skilled. I thought, "I know this feeling well from working on big projects myself." The only difference was that *I* was the project.

I felt fine coming out of the anaesthetic, happy that the surgery was over. I rested over the following weekend, and was not in much pain as long as I stayed in bed. I decided to return to work on Monday, but it was too early. I felt ill and nauseated, rather than feeling any pain at the point of incision. Originally I thought it was the side-effects of the anaesthetic that made me nauseated, but I believe that it was the effects of the actual surgery. I had to be careful not to lift anything for a few weeks.

Again, the diagnosis was non-cancerous. I felt lucky to be alive.

For a while I had a lot of scar tissue which felt at first like another lump and then like a ridge. The scar tissue from both surgeries has lessened considerably over time and has become almost imperceptible. Sometimes, especially in the first year, I felt an ache in my breast. These also have lessened over time. Because the incision was made on the underside of my left breast and went deep under it, there is little outward scarring.

Ever since my surgery, my annual mammograms take longer. Often I am called back in for another one. As with the second surgery and diagnosis, the fear of having breast cancer brings me back to the preciousness of life. I want to continue to live and celebrate my life in this awareness. I chose to be a part of this project because being photographed is about bringing my breasts into the light.

I feel huge relief that the lumps are non-cancerous, but the constant possibility also scares me. I feel as though I am an unwitting participant in a game of Russian roulette.

EDITOR'S NOTE: All the names in this story have been changed to protect the identity of the participant and her family.

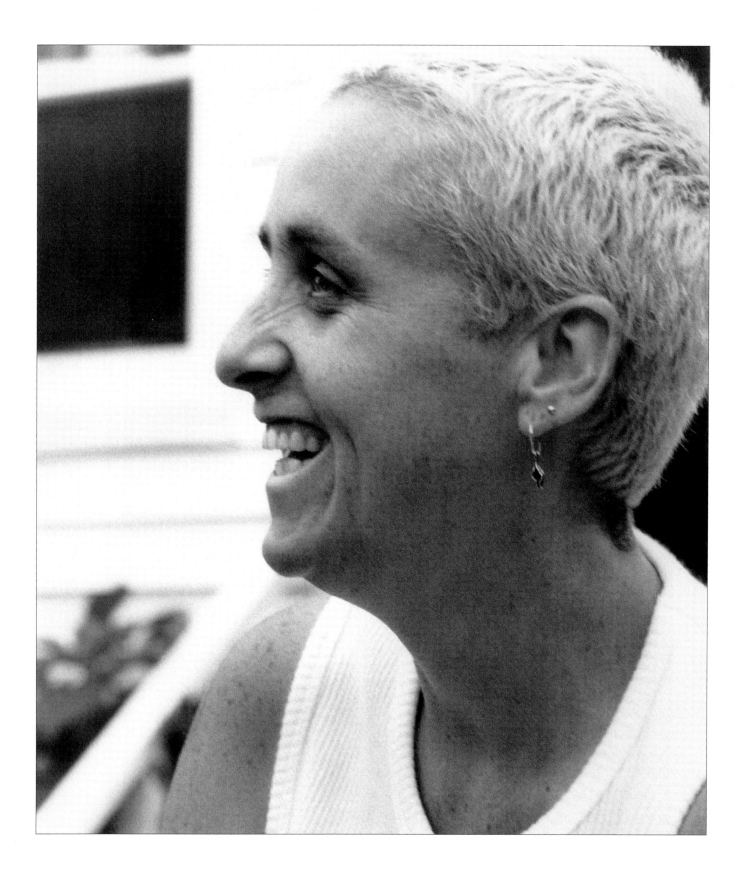

BOBBI AUBIN
Who's the Boss of My Body?

Bobbi Aubin's breast reduction surgery was a part of significant transformation in her life. Bobbi developed large breasts early as a girl and with them a high degree of self-consciousness about her body and sexuality, which contributed to her leaving school without graduating. She returned to high school in her mid-twenties, gave birth to a daughter, and began healing regarding childhood abuse experiences. In the course of this healing, she left an abusive marriage and lost a substantial amount of weight. It was at this time that she had her breasts reduced.

Bobbi is now employed as a Native child and family worker. She also teaches Wen-do (women's self-defense) and is involved in women's and lesbian rights activism in Sudbury.

Embarking on major life changes was not in my game plan. For a long time, I led my life according to the way my parents lived theirs. But then, that changed. Having breast reduction surgery was part of my coming into a new way of living. I am sharing my story for two reasons: for personal healing, and because I believe sharing life stories benefits others. I especially hope my story will help other women who are suffering.

I am of aboriginal ancestry. I am Métis. I grew up in a very small place in Northern Ontario called Windy Lake. For twenty-one years, we were the only family living there year-round. There were no neighbours, and therefore no kids to play with other than my own siblings. The French Catholic school that I attended was an hour away by bus. At school kids were forever calling me names — I felt different.

At first, I rebelled by shutting myself down and becoming a wallflower. I did it as a way to regain my self-worth. Growing up in physical isolation was difficult. I had no one I could trust or confide in. I kept everything inside, knowing and holding too many secrets. I also shut myself down because I was tired of being sexually and emotionally abused by one of my siblings. I started developing at a very early age. By the time I was nine years old, I had small breasts and had begun menstruating. I felt awkward; I was the only girl in my class who had breasts and was bleeding. All the girls and some of the boys in my class teased me constantly. I was a big tomboy. I hated having breasts. I wore baggy shirts to cover them up. I wanted to refuse to wear a bra, but my mother made me wear one. I was devastated about having to wear it. I hated being a girl.

When the students at my school began looking at me in a sexual way and teasing me, I felt even more uncomfortable in my body. Later I lashed out at them as a way to protect myself — I got kicked out of class so often that my high-school years were largely spent in and out of the principal's office. I eventually left without finishing high school.

In 1985 I met the man who was to be my husband for fifteen years. We moved in together shortly after we met, and things went downhill from there. Before I met him, I was as fit as fit could be from lifting weights and bicycling. But after I moved in with him, I started gaining weight and became very lazy. I stayed home, cooking all the "good foods" that my husband's Ukrainian mother liked to cook. I became the wife that my mother had been.

In about a year and a half, I ballooned up to three hundred pounds, and my breasts grew to 54 DD! They were so heavy that I could no longer wear a bra for support. The straps gouged grooves in my shoulders that were so painful I stopped wearing a bra. Eventually, gravity took over and my breasts became long and sore. That soreness continued throughout the following years, until I had reduction surgery.

After gaining so much weight, I felt unattractive and ashamed. Relatives made fun of my size all the time. I had low self-esteem and was miserable. When I told my husband that I was thinking of having my breasts reduced, he told me he'd divorce me if I did. That was in 1989. So I lived for a long time with the pain and shame of being very large-breasted. It wasn't until I left him in 1997 that I started to think again about a reduction.

After we were first married, my husband refused to let me work, so I decided to go back to high school. I was twenty-five. Throughout those years, and earlier, I hated sex, especially sex with my husband. Sometimes I think it's a miracle I ever got pregnant; but, during my last year of school, I became pregnant with my daughter, the only child I was to give birth to. My breasts remained the same size, and they were very painful during and after the pregnancy.

Looking back now, I see that I was very unhealthy, both physically and emotionally. I can see the path of self-destruction I was on. It had to change. After fif-teen years with my husband, I began to exercise again. I had been diagnosed with borderline diabetes, high cholesterol and high blood pressure. In order to get a handle on those health problems, I began walking the five miles along an old road till its end and back again. I also purchased a used bicycle and began riding it from the little northern town I was living in to another little town about fifteen miles away. I didn't lose weight right away, but the walking and biking helped me to escape and think logically.

In July 1997, I decided to tell my doctor about the incest I'd experienced as a child. I told him how unhappy I was. I told him I wanted to leave my marriage. My husband often drank heavily. I wanted to tell my husband about my experiences with incest, but I was brave enough to do that only when he was drunk. I found talking about my experiences with him enabling, but also frightening. His pattern was that at a certain point when he was drunk, he would begin to disbelieve me and would drink more. I began to feel afraid for my life. The day after I told my doctor about my fears, he took my daughter and me to a women's shelter in Sudbury where I was able to access service for our needs. That was July 15, 1997, and I have never looked back!

While I was at the shelter, I came out as a lesbian. I had lived my whole life in denial of my sexuality and by that time I had had enough. I came out full force, and immediately my body started to change. Within two months I went from 300 pounds to 140. I was not withdrawn anymore; I started living life as I should have been living it all along. I felt so much better emotionally, mentally and spiritually but the weight loss was too quick. My body changed drastically. My breasts stayed the same size, but became even longer — they hung down to my waist.

People noticed how unattractive they were. I tried not to let it bother me, but I could feel people staring.

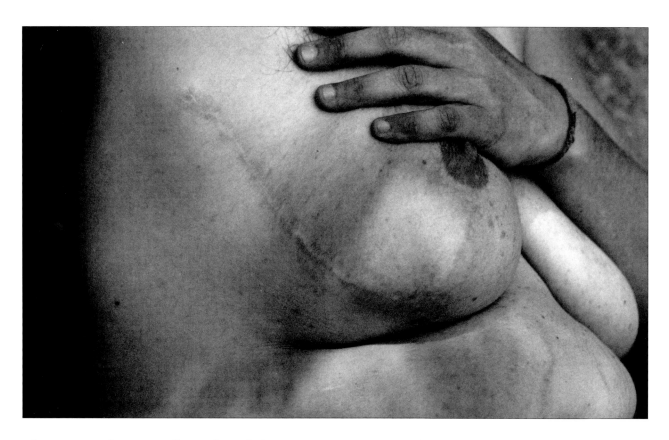

The surgeon who eventually performed the surgery described my breasts as "long, ropey, dangling masses." A woman once put her hands on my breasts, thinking they were my pregnant belly, and asked me when I was due. That hurt. I started college training in the Native Child and Family Worker program in 1999 and I noticed that my college classmates were nervous around me; I would hear comments in the halls. Although I joked about it with everyone, it really brought me down; I felt crushed. The worst thing was that all the women I met and were interested in were grossed out at the sight of me. The first woman I dated actually asked me to have my breasts reduced so we could have a better sex life, because she hated looking at them. I thought that if she saw me that way, then all

women would feel the same.

In 1999 I went back to see a doctor again because I was suffering from back pain. I chalked it up to being overweight, but when my doctor sent me for back x-rays, nothing showed up. That's when I started thinking about the weight of my breasts and how much they pulled downwards. Maybe they had been causing me all this pain. Then, in February 2000, I noticed that one of my nipples was discharging green fluid. I got really scared and went to see the school doctor. He sent me for a mammogram, which showed a large mass in my left breast. Luckily it turned out not to be cancer.

Knowing that mammograms were supposed to be painful procedures, other women asked me how it felt. I told them it had not hurt at all. I never felt it. The

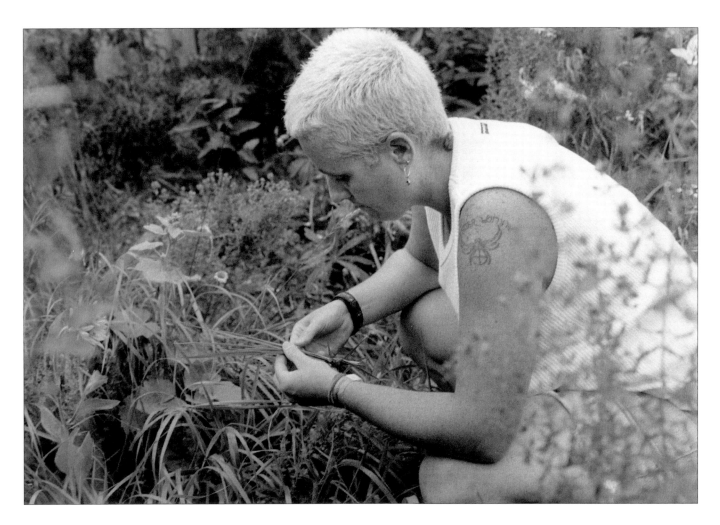

nurse attending the mammogram had been amazed at the weight of my breasts and also could not believe that I had no discomfort during the procedure. It turned out that the reason I did not feel any pain was that I had lost all sensation in my breasts because of their size and weight. The pain I had always associated with my breasts was in fact from the stretching of my skin.

I decided then and there that I would talk to a surgeon about breast reduction. That was in April 2000 and I was thirty-five years old. My physician called to make me an appointment to see a plastic surgeon. The surgeon that he called said he could not see me until December 2000, and then only for a consultation. If I were accepted for surgery, I would have to wait until April 2001! This was way too long a wait, so I took the reins in my own hands and called another surgeon. Within two weeks I was in his office. When he examined me, he told me he couldn't believe I had gone this long with my breasts the way they were. He told me about the surgery, the procedure and the complications. He also told me that he performed over five hundred breast reductions a year. We talked for a long time and I felt really comfortable with him. Within another two weeks, I had been approved by OHIP and was scheduled for breast reduction surgery.

By May I was sitting in the hospital waiting room. There were two other women there that day for other reasons; one had her mother with her and one had her sister with her. They were scared. When they asked what I was having done, I told them about my breasts. They were very sympathetic. They asked who was there to support me and I had to tell them that no one had come. They asked where my mother was. I told them that she did not know I was having surgery, and neither did the rest of my family. (I haven't seen or spoken with my family since I disclosed the abuse that I had experienced and came out as a lesbian.) The mother started to cry when I told her this and I told her I was okay. She hugged me before I went in. I will never forget her.

The surgeon came and took me into a preparation room. With a big permanent marker, he began drawing lines on my chest where he would make cuts and remove tissue. I felt a little silly sitting there with lines all over my breasts. He asked me what size I wanted them to be. I told him to make them as small as possible and that I was serious! I looked down at my breasts, knowing this would be the last time I would ever see them. I couldn't wait till it was over. I was wheeled into the operating room and put under.

When I woke up, there was a policewoman sitting on my bed — an incredible sight to wake up to! She is a straight friend of mine who knows I love women in uniform, so she decided to come and see me while she was still on duty. She was the perfect person to wake up to.

After the usual hug and chat, I looked down at my chest and was amazed at the sight. My chest was wrapped in gauze and a tensor bandage, and there were no bulges hanging over my belly or to the sides of my chest. Before the surgery, whenever I lay down, my breasts would slide off my chest and rest under my armpits. My ex-husband used to call them "water wings."

I had gone in for surgery huge-breasted and had woken up with part of me missing. I thought I would be sad at the loss, but I was quite relieved. I started to cry, not because I had lost my breasts, but because I felt lighter and almost pain-free. The physical relief I felt was immediate. Even weeks after the surgery, I did not mind the small, stinging pain that remained. The entire procedure was far less painful than what I had experienced during all those years before the surgery. I went from a size 54DD bra to a large sports bra. It felt great no longer to have the heaviness of my breasts.

Some time after the surgery, I ran into my first female lover, the one who had had the issue about my breasts. She noticed immediately that I was smaller. When I told her I had had the surgery, she said it had been her influence over me. I told her I had done it on my own and for myself only. She then had the nerve to ask me out. I blatantly told her to fuck off!

This surgery has had a tremendous impact on my self-esteem and sense of self-worth. For many years I had told myself it shouldn't matter what a person looks like, but when I began to suffer in all aspects of my life, I decided I had had enough. Taking care of myself by having a reduction allowed me to become a more balanced physical, mental, emotional and spiritual being. I am happy and healthy today. I no longer smoke, I have almost finished my college course, and I am pursuing a career in social work. No one is ever going to tell me what I can or cannot do with my body again. I own myself — and I love who I am. Who's the boss of my body? … I am!

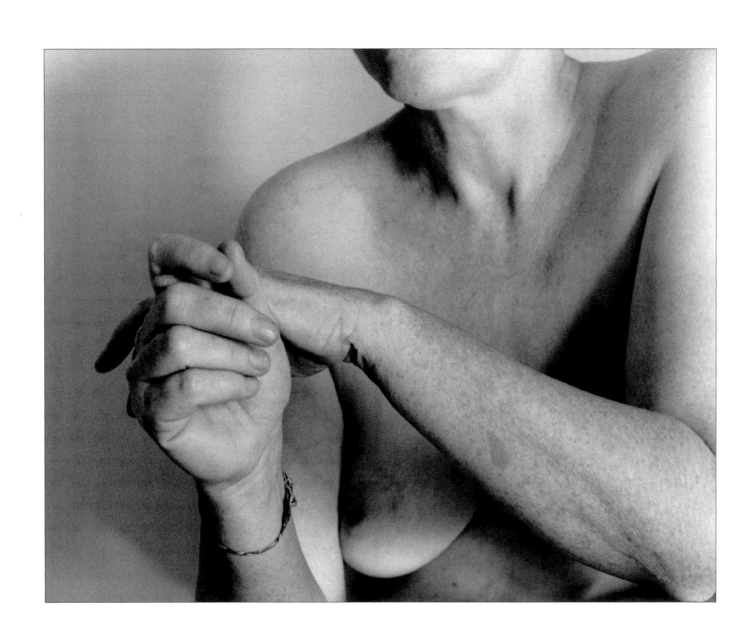

NANCY VIVA DAVIS HALIFAX
This Tissue is Memory (Poem)

Nancy Viva Davis Halifax went for breast reduction surgery at the age of forty-two to reduce pain related to large breasts after having breast-fed two daughters. The pathology reports on the tissue removed showed cancer previously undetected by self-examinations or mammogram. Nancy initially was considering radiation treatment but then opted for mastectomy.

Nancy is a visual artist and poet, and has recently completed her PhD in Arts-Informed Research at the Ontario Institute for Studies in Education. Nancy's doctoral work was radically changed through her participation in My Breasts, My Choice. *Her poetic transcription for the project formed the base for her arts-driven thesis. Nancy is a Post-Doctoral Fellow at the University Health Network, University of Toronto, where she is representing research in the field of cancer education using poetics and the arts.*

VULNERABILITY INCARNATE

Incarnate.
Clotted
red vowels
of beginnings.
A history buried under
dirt.
A bloody word
making weeds of
flower and flesh.

Life is full of vulnerability.
Imagine being split open
your whole being open to the world as it passes
the world passes through you,
even the birds
neglect the dreamer.

A bird interrupts its flighty reverie —
stands over you
throws your
corrugated cardboard of muscle and bone
into relief.

The relief of shadow.
In imagination shadow'd vulnerable being
cherishes luminescence,
the scent of the lost,
the luminescence of skinned ideas.
Life is full of vulnerability.
Leave aside
what you cannot account for,
leave familiar tales.
Don't tell me about bias.
Clinical objectivity is fully worn.

FIRST QUARTER

at thirteen

I remember my breath under lazy trees,
uphill tumbling into a half-opened world,
white t-shirted days.

I remember the gingered
awkward body freckled from sun
pale and translucent
skin bordering
vellum
before the first mark is made.

SECOND QUARTER

at nineteen (motor vehicle accident)

I
screamin', bone crackin', distanced
fleshed, skinned
severed at nineteen
and when her eyes opened
one at a time
she was split to the world.
The goddess in bestowing her grace
harnessed my body to her
wheels till my rims buckled.
Hurled my limbs
through space into night
lit by car lights.

Darkness
brakes
over my fallen body.
The witnesses to my final flight
fire
flies

II
What is the opposite of an angel?
For that is what I am.

She was never an angel. She stepped off the cliff
    without wings
and landed a cripple. Not even scars where wings
might once have been. Beside her on the pavement a
mouse has been born in the fractures of the sidewalk.
Smaller than her baby fingernail the feet are grey
fronds of sacred artemisia. This youngling lies quietly
on her side and I beside her, my head on earth
hope withers.
I see her chest no longer blossoms.

The girl who is
not a blessed one
born into life
screamin' crimson
disappears me —
demands, takes over.
Bound together —
I scream at her when there is no-one close to us.
Few know of her.
I fill my arms with her body
and she sleeps.

Sighs
the plush caress of
flesh
slays me

I betray her
by a wince, a flatness in my voice.
Clouds grey my speech.
A dove
sodden cardboard
leaves fluttering
wings, cooing and
wings will not stay.
I am an aerialist
flapping at ground level,
fogged in.

III

When she is first born I do not know how to care for her.
An only child, and I do not favour her. My hand lingers on greyhound ribs.
She suffers terribly. There are days when she cannot get up and I am tender with her. I worry that if our sisterhood be found out we will be abandoned. Neither loved.

IV

I wake up early to bake scones for her breakfast,
hot coffee and jam and butter wander down the stairs
to knock at her door.
She is not able to eat what I cook.
On some days turns her head
and the bones of her back tell me.

I worry.
I lean my head against her door
listen
I hear red and blue whispers.
Dreamt a ward filled with twenty-three other beds
a long, narrow room with pale yellow walls of curtains.
Veiled windows loose coarse moans.
Each bed grips its own ruined secret.

The bird stands close to me
golden-eyed and
just beyond the
stillness
of shadow.

V

There is no straight and narrow endurance
within my body
coloured gestures of stone
hunger toward a dim light
where letters coupled and singly
mate conceiving the never-yet-worded.
At the end of this line
a cadmium red stands
small and stark against a salty cobalt.
One on top the other.

VI

Remember you are at the edge of the ordinary. Once
through those doors your world of meaning vanishes.
Walk across the yard now,
through the half-melted dun snow,
sink down

and up the stairs of the sanctuary.
Ruins
stain your body
incarnadine.

THIRD QUARTER

night bus (biopsy)

I
Mid-January.
Snow moves the horizon.
Dawn steadies me in half-light.

II
I take a taxi to the hospital.
I could have boarded the night bus.
Fluorescent bright with a driver
who speaks with great assurance
as he names stops:
Dundas West, Symington, Lansdowne, Dufferin,
Dovercourt, Ossington, Christie.
On the bus a man sits too close. Lies back on his seat
with legs apart, his hands between his thighs. He looks
at–through me, body–me.
A detour announced
the passengers need reassurance.
The driver is calm and clearly repeats:
This bus will proceed south on Spadina until
*   Harbord Street*
at which point we will continue east
until we reach St. George Street
at that point we will travel north

until we meet Bloor Street where we will continue south
along the established route.
Passenger
passenger after passenger walks the aisle of the bus to
ask the same question.
The forms
shaven, querulous, authoritative, anxious, unwashed.
Missed steps are sounded as
the bus driver and I swerve.

II
Laced black boots fumble the buttons of my coat.
No coffee.
The list of do's
the cotton comfort of socks and black-and-white
striped long johns
during surgery.
I open my door, close and lock it.
The stairs are covered with snowshoed flakes,
who do not linger as
my stride through half-light
takes me to the end of my street to
hail a taxi.
My steps fade into icicled silence.
The taxi man who stops is brown and the sounds of
    his car are warm.

III
The taxi man asks me where I am going.
I tell him my destination and huddle against the door.
I am quiet.
Listen to our breaths harmonize to the hum of the
*   radio dispatch.*

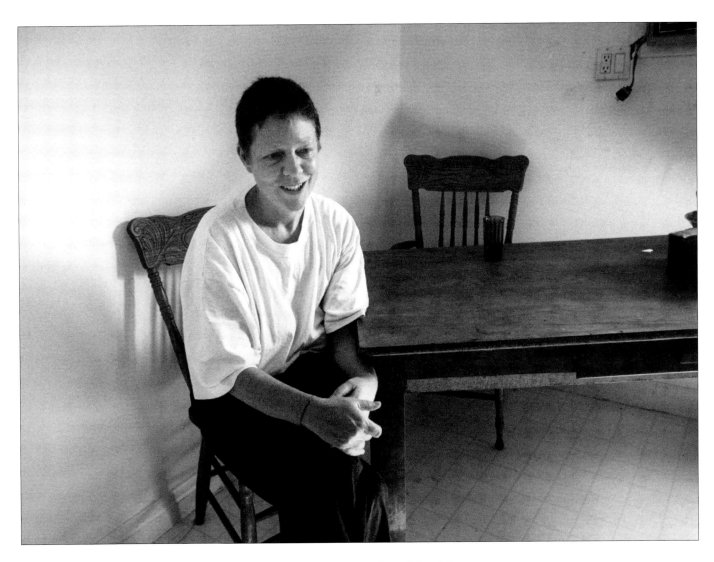

We continue until the radiant chorus of falling snow
melts our road.

IV
Speech relinquished. The warmth of bodies
the pulse of our blood as we drive together, ends when
we stop
and the taxi man turns to me:
Seven dollars.
I give the taxi man ten dollars

though he drives me
to a place where I do not
want to arrive.

V
I don't know how to protect myself anymore.
A pill sticks in my throat.
I saw a squirrel today.
a wet glove dropped by the road. Its legs
finger sleeves, its tail
a thumb cozy.

And where I would insert my hand
that is where there is no head.

VI
The hallway is cold. Cold rooms
inhabited by machines
unbearable positions.

Hold, they say.   How?   I wonder.
Don't breathe.
Whispers
of unseen light pass through my body,
soft-spoken light.
Is that what they want me to be?
Soft-edged drawn desire
pleasures of pleasing
I cannot conjure that girl into existence
yet I do not cry out.
I spare the other her vulnerability.

VII
Along these corridors
the sound of my walking is not heard,
the not sound of my walking aches,
ground delight dissolves.
A bed with wheels carries my body.
Hear steps of the faded green moving me
smell wheels, smell doors.

FOURTH QUARTER

a woman is told

I
Described by a man she does not know,
translated by icy, certain words
she becomes "a case."
A new vocabulary marks her.

abnormality biopsy carcinoma
dissection excision fascia haemostasis
intercostobrachial lesion lymph
plexus rectus subdermal
thoracodural vascular weal.

She sits in a chair, cross-legged, drinking cold coffee
the tips of her fingers trace the blind fault between
        her eyes.
She doesn't cry until the surgeon calls her
wee lamb.
Tears
singe the floor of a room
where dust floats
down.
Feet rustle in paper slippers the colour of
her first tattoos
(four blue periods
ending sentences
murmured in a dim room
where lasers
target that swell).

II
Rough, sterile cloth drapes
her breast
for its last appearance.
She traces the pulse of blood through veins
under translucent skin.
Her breast
is vellum for the calligraphy of the surgeon
a sampler for the stitches of a new resident
an artefact for the pathologist.
The first line appears
colours bleed
scarlet lake, rose madder.

III
She walks into the pathology department
unchallenged
by the white coats.
Sees tissue in freezers
stained, sectioned, sliced
remembers
her breast.
It was warm.
She wants to feel
she tells herself.
It's not just a mastectomy.
The pulse of memory is cauterized,
ivory skin memory
warmed by breath, kissed by shadow.
Not just a breast rests
in the gloved hand of the surgeon
This tissue
is memory.

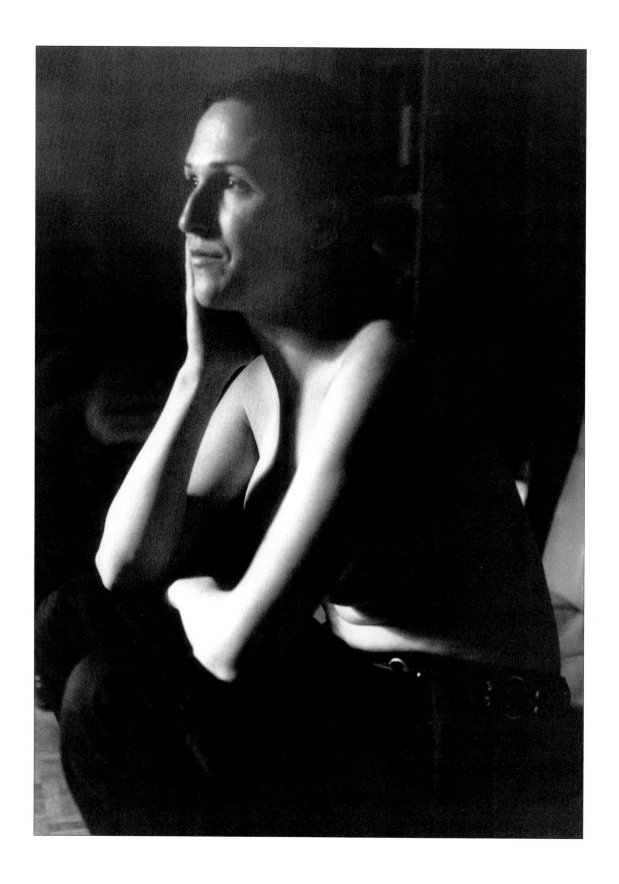

Mirha-Soleil Ross
Negotiating Choice

Although Mirha-Soleil Ross was labelled a biological male at birth, the development of breasts in early adolescence and other gender-crossing characteristics left her caught somewhere in between boy and girl. At sixteen Mirha-Soleil decided to live as male and pursued mastectomy for complete breast tissue removal. At twenty, she chose to live more truly to her sense of self and began living as a woman. At thirty, she had her first breast augmentation surgery with saline implants. Her left breast turned out "perfect," her right breast encapsulated — the breast was hard, the augmentation too high, and she lost a significant amount of sensation in her right breast area. To have these issues corrected, Mirha-Soleil had to decide whether to return to the same surgeon (which reduced costs for her), or pursue an alternative surgeon (a highly expensive endeavor). She returned to the first surgeon. The encapsulation was addressed, however the implant still remained high. A third surgery to correct this was only partially successful. Mirha-Soleil is hoping for improvement through further surgery.

Mirha-Soleil is a Toronto-based videographer, performance artist, and radical animal rights and sex workers' activist. She is interviewed by My Breasts, My Choice *editor Barbara Brown.*

Mirha-Soleil: I've been through two breast surgeries so far and it looks like I'm heading for at least two more.

I had my first breast surgery, a mastectomy, when I was sixteen years old. That surgery was part of a desperate attempt to pass and live as a boy and hopefully to bloom as a human being. My medical history is tortuously simple: I was born with a penis (albeit petite and overly circumcised) and testicles, so I was assigned the sex "male" and the gender "boy." But, from as far back as I can remember, I exhibited both behavioural and physical traits that contradicted this classification. I was an overly "emotional" child and teenager, crying like a sissy all the time. I didn't have any interest in playing hockey with boys, and especially not with their dirty trucks. I had a very high-pitched voice, which gained me the nickname "the Whistle" in school and among my family. I didn't look, move, talk, scream or breathe like a boy, and wasn't able to interact with the world as a boy. I wasn't able to get the world to see me, read me or treat me like a boy. Therefore I wasn't socialized as a boy. I sometimes wonder if I was ever socialized at all!

To top it all off, my breasts started to grow out of nowhere when I was ten years old. I didn't end up with a C cup, but my titties ended up being way too big for what a young, skinny boy should have had. I will spare you a detailed account of the harassment and violence I endured as a child who had been ordered to — but couldn't — pass as a boy. Suffice it to say that at some point, enough became enough, and I felt my only way to survive was to make drastic changes to my body, my physical appearance, my voice and my mannerisms in order to pass and function as a boy. I knew I wasn't going to be able to pass as a masculine straight man, so I constructed for myself a nice little androgynous, extroverted, queer boy character. I was attracted to men, but I knew that I couldn't be eroticized as a boy by gay boys if they felt some titties were going on when we went to bed. So removing my breasts became imperative in order to fulfill my desire for social and sexual integration as a boy in the queer community.

A lot of people wrongly assume that, because I am a transsexual, I was once a "man" and became a "woman." I think most people, including other transsexual women and men, have difficulty grasping what my experience with social transition and physical transformation was like. They're used to having people changing clearly from male to female, or vice versa. I don't think they see that my mastectomy was a necessary step in my transition towards living and being accepted as a male. It's weird for me to be classified as a male-to-female transsexual. It does not reflect the sex and gender transformations I have been through. What I went through was a transition from "something-girlish-in-between" to male, and then from androgynous boy to female. This idea is difficult to understand because people, even most transsexuals, can only understand what is in the realm of their own experience.

BARBARA: You refer to your first surgery as a mastectomy. What's the difference between a mastectomy and a reduction in this situation?

MIRHA-SOLEIL: I've always called it a mastectomy because that's how the doctors referred to it at the time. From what I gather, they used to call it a reduction when they reduced the breast mass but didn't completely remove the breast tissue. With a reduction, they didn't try to make you look like you never had breasts at all. I call what I had a mastectomy because the goal of it was to get my tits chopped off.

BARBARA: Did you have family or friends supporting you through the decision-making process?

MIRHA-SOLEIL: No, I had nobody at all who supported me. It was quite an awful process. For my parents, just as for me, there was a lot of shame around my being feminine, having a girl voice, and having grown breasts. My mother was in denial about it all, even though at the same time she was constantly struggling to prove to people everywhere that I was a boy. People would respond, "If he's a boy, how come he's got boobs?" Our family doctor, whom we consulted every two months during my teenage years, used to tell us it was normal for a certain percentage of the male teenage population to grow breasts, that it was called gynaecomastia, and that my breasts would most likely go away as I got older. This family doctor used to tell me, "Don't worry, you won't become a homosexual because you're growing breasts. And people harass you in school because they're jealous." I used to find his comments very peculiar, because I really couldn't picture any of my macho male bullies dying for a pair of tits!

I kept on insisting we go back to see the doctor, so my mother and I repeated our visits to him more frequently. He eventually got tired of us and referred us to an endocrinologist, who realized there was indeed a problem and who referred us to a plastic surgeon. Even though I was extremely traumatized by the idea of having to go to hospital, having someone cut through my nipples and rip my flesh apart, I was determined to improve my quality of life. I had already dropped out of school because the harassment and beatings that had occurred on a daily basis for almost ten years had become too much. So living as a boy with a boy's body was serious business for me.

There was a lot of discussion in Quebec at the time, in the newspapers and on television, about women who had had their lives ruined by botched cosmetic surgeries. One very outspoken victim of these botched surgeries was Rachel Boutin, founder and spokesperson for L'Association des opérés en chirurgie esthétique (L'ADOCE). Her organization provides information about the different types of cosmetic surgeries available as well as referrals to responsible, reputable surgeons. So I made an appointment with Rachel Boutin.

The first thing she does when meeting someone is assess whether or not the person's desire for surgery is reasonable. I went to her office. She sat behind her desk, lit a cigarette, and asked me to take my top off. I removed my three layers of shirts. When she looked at my tits, she seemed a bit taken back and said, "Definitely these have got to go!" It was very validating and empowering to finally have someone sympathize so strongly with me and understand my desire to get rid of my breasts. She took out her referral notepad and gave me the name and number of a guy she considered to be an excellent surgeon; he worked out of an English-speaking hospital and taught cosmetic surgery at a local university.

My only real dilemma was to justify my decision to have breast surgery, given my commitment to animal rights. I was very involved in the animal rights movement at that age. I was strongly critical of the pharmaceutical and medical establishments; I resented the idea that these men, who most likely had tortured and killed animals as part of their medical training, would be touching my body. These doctors and medical institutions represented a system and stood by a set of ethics that I opposed, so I resented them receiving money as a result of my choices. I was very unhappy about the idea of having to take painkillers after surgery, because they would have been tested on animals and might contain animal products. I had to do some deep thinking and reach an understanding with-

in myself that this was the context and paradigm within which I, and the people working in the medical system, were stuck — that my going ahead with this surgery didn't have to contradict my views about animal experimentation as a useless and vicious waste of taxpayers' dollars. I decided to go ahead with it.

When I was young, hospitals gave me the creeps, made me feel very anxious and nauseous, so I wasn't looking forward to my stay there. I was scared that I might suffer a total breakdown and cry all the time. But I didn't do badly at all, emotionally speaking. The hospitalization was a little difficult because the staff at the hospital didn't speak French and I could only babble a few words in English. So much for Canada and Quebec being bilingual places where you can receive basic essential services in both French and English! To help me understand their questions during the pre-surgery examinations, the interns and nurses made clumsy drawings of a bladder, kidney, liver and testicle on a piece of paper. The most awkward event was when the surgeon brought in his plastic-surgery students and made me undress and stand in front of them. He gave them a lecture about my case and what he was going to do with me, and used a black marker to make convoluted circles around my chest — all of that in English, of course, so I couldn't understand a word of what they were discussing. I felt like a "really interesting French case!"

I should mention that the surgeon used what is referred to as the "keyhole technique" to remove my breast tissue. This technique is used to remove breasts that are not bigger than an A cup. He made an incision in the lower part of my nipples, an incision that extended outwards to just over a centimetre on each side. He did what would be considered a very good job at the time. But I've met quite a few female-to-male transsexuals who have had the same technique used on them in recent years and all of them had the incision around the areola instead of inside the nipples, and their scars were much less visible than mine. The provincial health plan in Quebec covered my surgery because they considered it a medical necessity.

BARBARA: How was the aftermath? What was the healing process like?

MIRHA-SOLEIL: I was hospitalized for five days. I had a drain on the side of each breast for most of that time. I was hooked up to an intravenous for two days and, throughout my body, I felt pretty wrecked. When I woke up from the surgery, I was quite shocked by the size of my chest. With the dressings and the swelling, my breasts looked four times bigger than they had before the surgery. When they removed the dressings, my breasts were blue, purple, yellow, black and red and as hard as if the doctors had implanted metallic balloons under my skin.

The recovery and healing process was long, very long. After the five days in hospital, I spent two weeks in bed at home and one month barely able to move around. My chest looked horrible — bruised and swollen — for at least one month. The scars from the incisions and where they placed the drains were also puffy and swollen for a very long time. It actually took over a year before all the swelling went away and I started to have something that looked like a normal chest. I say "something like" because, even though I ended up being flat-chested, my chest always felt and looked a bit odd in my own eyes. I was always a bit self-conscious about not having a "natural" male chest.

BARBARA: After the surgery, was there a shift in people's attitudes towards you?

MIRHA-SOLEIL: As I mentioned, I had already dropped out of school, which was the main place outside of my family where people knew I had breasts. Outside of school, I had become very good at concealing my breasts, so most people didn't know I'd had surgery. For example, I had started working with an alternative theatre group and no one in the group knew that I had breasts. I'd always been scared that the teacher in the group would one day ask us to remove our shirts or have us wear an undershirt for exercises. Then, one month after my surgery, we had a summer party, and for the first time I told everyone about my titties' history. I even showed everyone my scars and bruising. Even though people thought this was a horrible sight — I looked like a diesel truck had run over my chest — I felt completely comfortable showing them my body, something I would never have considered just one month before. It was so liberating!

BARBARA: So in terms of your movement from having the mastectomy to going out into your life and living as a boy . . .

MIRHA-SOLEIL: I started to be more outgoing, and I felt a little more self-confident. I started to wear t-shirts. I started to consider experimenting sexually. I was not comfortable enough to start having sex with anyone, though, until I was maybe eighteen or nineteen. I had lots of other body and gender issues going on. There were other parts of my body that I couldn't and didn't want to change. For example, I couldn't and didn't want to stretch and make my dick bigger or build my muscles to fit the macho standards of the gay male community even though it was the one I wanted to be a part of. I was only able and willing to do so much, emotionally and physically, to try to fit into that scene.

BARBARA: So from there, did you find a way in? Acceptance or not? Was it easy to enter into the gay community?

MIRHA-SOLEIL: My background is filled with experiences of my being harassed, violated, and beaten as a child and a teenager. I come from a place of deep hurt and pain. When I decided that I was going to live as a queer boy, I naively thought my experiences were typical, and I expected other boys in the queer community to share my history of daily harassment and violence. I expected them to be tolerant, open-minded, sensitive, understanding, compassionate people as a result of all the shit I assumed they also must have gone through. But I found out that a lot of gay men were and always had been masculine guys who had it easy as kids and who sometimes were the sort of bullies who beat up on me. I found out that the gender and sexual repression and the violence I had endured were not common experiences amongst most gay men. I also found out quite rapidly that gay men were primarily attracted to hyper-masculine, straight-acting men with big muscles and big dicks, and I didn't fit that description in any way. I found out that the queer community was just as oppressive and repressive as any other group of people when it came to sex, gender, and body diversity. I found out that my body and who I was were not sexually "marketable" in the gay male community. Even the other femme boys whom I was attracted to were self-deprecating; they drooled in front of these pseudo-straight clowns, instead of developing a critical analysis of the gender- and body-based repression that exists within the mainstream North American gay male culture. So, at the age of twenty, after four years of masquerading and attempting to live up to the standards of masculinity in the queer community, I came to the conclusion that I would never be able to integrate completely in society as a boy. I accepted that, as a boy, I couldn't relate to other boys or men sexually, emotionally, psychologically, spiritually, or politically. So I decided to revert back to my original feminine sex and gender self.

From the age of sixteen to twenty, I wanted to pass as a boy; then from twenty on, I decided that I wanted to pass unambiguously as a woman. I grew up being an "in-between" and that no longer interested me from a personal, practical or political point of view. Especially now, as I'm growing older, I have no interest in being or adopting a third, fourth, or fifth sex or gender or anything like that. I don't identify as transgendered and I object to some inherently anti-transsexual stances that permeate North American, English-speaking transgender politics. But that doesn't mean that as a woman, I now conform 100 percent to female gender expectations or will try to erase from my body and myself all traces of my sex and gender history.

BARBARA: What are these traces?

MIRHA-SOLEIL: I have a little Adam's apple, for example, and I find it is very charming, even sexy, so I wouldn't get rid of it. At this point, I just wouldn't want to change my body completely. The same androgynous qualities that I enjoyed having when living as a boy I now enjoy as a woman. The stuff I'm interested in changing is obvious stuff: breasts and genitals.

BARBARA: And you've recently made more choices about breast surgery.

MIRHA-SOLEIL: Yes. Depending on whichever sex and gender I am living with, I always feel that my primary and secondary sex characteristics are inadequate. When I was living as a boy, my penis looked underdeveloped. When I began living as a woman, my breasts felt and looked too small. I always felt as if I had either a childish penis or childish, perky titties. I got to a point where my external sex characteristics — primarily my breasts and my penis — did not reflect who I felt I was inside. I'm in my thirties now and I want my genitals and my breasts to reflect that age. I didn't want to become a forty year old woman with twelve year old looking titties. And I hope I won't become a fifty year old woman with a twelve year old looking penis! So my decision to get breast implants didn't have that much to do with being a transsexual. It didn't have much to do with being comfortable with intimacy either, as I am lucky to have a very sweet male partner. I've been living with him for four years and he is very accepting, even appreciative, of my physical "irregularities."

BARBARA: And what are people's attitudes towards you, now that you have had the surgery?

MIRHA-SOLEIL: I'm a sex worker, and the number of men who want to spend time with me has definitely increased. Men do like substantial breasts, there's no doubt about that, but they are quite flexible in terms of what these substantial breasts can look like. I have a certain number of guys I was scared to lose because I know they enjoyed my small breasts, but they've adapted to my bigger ones. Obviously they weren't just sticking around with me because I had cute tiny titties.

Living as a woman, first with a penis and unusually small breasts, and now with the results of a boob job gone bad, has made me realize how open-minded and tolerant straight men are in terms of the types of women's bodies they're ready to get it on with. We always hear feminists whine all over the damn place about how heterosexual men objectify women, reduce them to pussies and tits, etc. According to the sacred texts of feminism, men have narrow visions of which female bodies are socially and sexually acceptable or beautiful.

I don't know where these feminists live or how many men they've slept with. I am especially curious about the specific cultural, ethnic and linguistic backgrounds of the men they interviewed for their surveys, because my experience of sleeping with countless straight men contradicts what they say. Ninety percent of the men I see as a sex worker are South Asian, African, Italian, Portuguese, Arabic, Greek, Latino, French, and come from a working-class background. I don't have a very significant White Anglo and middle-class following. Most of my clients are actually construction workers — that is also my family's background — and my overall experience with them has been enlightening and sexually validating. They are turned on by all kinds of women — fat women, skinny women, women with cellulite — and for them a pair of tits is a pair of tits! Whether they're saggy, flat, or pointing in wild directions — give them those tits and they'll suck on them like there's no tomorrow. Everything I've presumed about straight men's openness to a diversity of women's bodies, including a diversity of breast shapes and sizes, has been confirmed since I got my breast implants.

As far as I'm concerned, my right breast feels like a rock and it is literally deformed. I have developed severe scar encapsulation — a build-up of scar tissue — around my right implant. It's too high, which makes my nipple look like it's running away under my breast. And yet I haven't had any guy say anything demeaning or hurtful about it; rather it's the opposite. They tell me I have beautiful breasts.

BARBARA: So your experience stands in opposition to what we could call popular culture imagery. Because I do think there is an image published in papers and magazines that prescribes a particular look, a very limited image of beauty. And there's a fight against

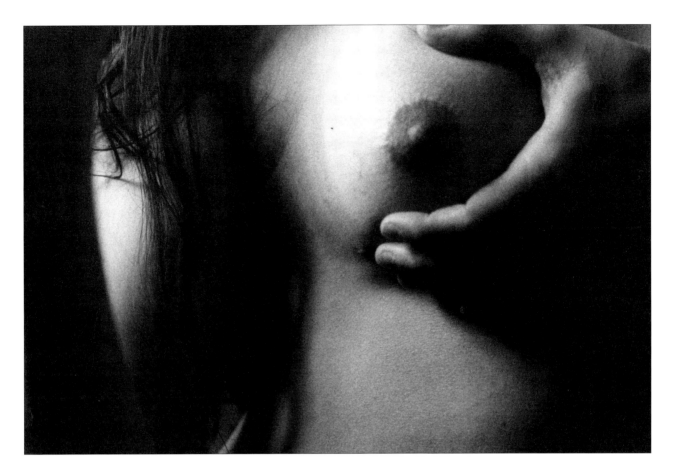

that. But what I hear you saying is that there is a lived reality that indicates that men's acceptance of beauty is larger than what's published.

MIRHA-SOLEIL: Yes, and that's because the majority of men do not sleep with those women we see in fashion and porno magazines, in *Playboy,* etc. Those women — skinny, with a small frame, petite ass, firm and perky breasts, perfect skin — might be the ones we see in popular culture imagery and in the media, and men do fantasize about sleeping with those women, but the reality is that most women do not look like that. So men's lived sexual experiences are with fat women, women who have cellulite, breasts in all directions, large asses, bushy genitals, and pimples. And, as I said earlier, we come from various ethnic, cultural and geo-graphical backgrounds, so we don't all share the same references and standards of beauty. I, for example, come from a Québecois, working-class and poor back-ground and the women that men are used to loving and living and sleeping with in that context are dif-ferent from the ones that White, Anglo middle-class guys are used to. French, Québecois, working-class men are more used to dealing with strong, grounded, loud, and sexually assertive women who won't put up with men who won't eat their pussy!

So I guess there are two overlapping phenomena going on. The first one is, if men's sexual experiences with women are with those who do not fit stereo-typical ideals of beauty, then it makes sense that, if they're going to spend fifteen bucks on a magazine, or five bucks on a video, or 150 bucks on an escort, they will probably want to experience something different from what they're used to experiencing in their everyday lives. They might want to buy images of women who don't look like their wives and girlfriends because they're curious and want to try something else.

The second one is that many guys complain about being bored with what is offered by the porn industry. There is a growing demand for alternative and amateur porn, of videos showing people fucking and sucking each other in their basements. When you look at these porn films, they are real people with real bodies, bellies and pimples. The fact that these videos are more and more popular is, I think, a sign that there are a lot of men and a growing number of women who want to see that — who want to see themselves reflected in sexual imagery.

BARBARA: They are seeking some kind of integrity between their experience and the images they get to consume.

MIRHA-SOLEIL: Yes. A lot of men and women find it a turn-on to see people with bodies that look real, bodies that they can identify as familiar, everyday bodies. Because often those are the bodies they are most likely to encounter and have sex with, as opposed to encountering Pamela Anderson, whom they can only fantasize about.

BARBARA: When you decided to have breast augmentation surgery, what was your process for finding a surgeon?

MIRHA-SOLEIL: I spoke with all the transsexual women I knew who had breast implants. I asked them all kinds of questions. What type of implants did they have put in, textured or smooth? Where was the incision — under the arms, around the nipple, in the belly but-

ton? What was the size of the implants in relation to how many ccs of saline water was put in them? How much breast development or tissue did they have before the surgery? Did they have any complications? Encapsulation? Deflation? How much did they pay? How arrogant was their plastic surgeon (because many of them seem to be)? I asked tons of questions. And then I tried to figure out what I wanted for myself. I made appointments with two surgeons. One charged the average price, $5,000, and claimed he had done the largest number of breast surgeries in the entire country. The other one was this upscale, top-of-the-line surgeon who has an impeccable reputation, worked mostly for wealthy and glamorous people, and charged almost $8,000. They both gave simplistic "written-in-advance" answers to my questions and tried to get rid of me as soon as possible. The upscale surgeon charged me $160 for a six-minute consultation.

I decided to go for the cheaper one because, with him, any post-surgical problem, such as scar encapsulation, would be paid for. The rich one said nothing would be covered. And I couldn't afford the $8,000 he was asking.

The price of my surgery, $4,800, covered the hospital, the anaesthesiologist, the surgeon's fees, and the implants. I got a loan from a financing institution in Vancouver that specializes in providing fast money for folks who have expensive vet or medical bills. I didn't like my surgeon's demeanour when I consulted with him, but a plastic surgeon is a plastic surgeon. I believe in judging a surgeon by his reputation and by looking at the work she or he has done before. The five transsexual women I knew who'd had their surgeries done by him had very nice, soft, natural-looking breasts.

One of the most important things I was looking for in a surgeon was an openness to discussing options in terms of the size of the implants, the placement of the incision, and whether the implant was going to be on top of or under the pectoral muscle. I find that most surgeons follow certain trends when it comes to these options. Most of them right now, for example, will not consider putting the implant on top of the muscle. Some will insist that it should be a specific size, usually too big. And then they will give us obscure reasons why it should be their way. I find that, in most cases, the decisions they make for us regarding all of these choices derive from their own personal preferences and professional biases, which they then try to present as scientifically based. And how can you argue with them? They are the experts! This particular surgeon, however, was open to exploring different options for me, so that was a big point in his favour when the time came to choose who was going to operate on me.

BARBARA: What was the reason behind choosing to have the implants put on top of the muscle?

MIRHA-SOLEIL: The five transsexual women I mentioned did have their breast implants put on top of the muscle and they had very soft, natural-looking and -feeling breasts — breasts that will sag with time. I wanted breasts like that. Most transsexual women who had their implants put under the muscle, by other surgeons, had very firm and, in some cases, hard breasts. But the ones who had them put on top of the muscle were also fatter than I am and had at least a big B cup before augmentation, whereas most of the ones who had their implants put under the muscle had nothing more than an A cup before. For implants placed on top of the muscle, having significant breast tissue between the skin and the implants helps to make the breasts feel more natural. I had very little breast tissue but I still wanted the implants on top, even though I didn't know how they'd turn out.

These kinds of issues are the ones that the doctors are not prepared to fully explore with us. They don't treat us as intelligent people. They are either offensive in their attempts to confuse us with medical jargon or they give us answers that are condescending in their simplicity.

BARBARA: You spoke about the aftermath of your mastectomy. What was it like after your breast augmentation in terms of pain, discomfort and the healing process?

MIRHA-SOLEIL: With the mastectomy I felt like a tank had run me over. After the augmentation I was in pain for only a few days — nothing compared to the intensity of the mastectomy. And the pain and bruising went away quite fast. A week after the surgery, I appeared naked in some erotic scenes for *G-SPrOuT!*, an experimental video about veganism and sexuality that my boyfriend and I were preparing for a film festival. I participated in some sexually explicit scenes with my stitches still in. Cutting flesh from a breast is different from inserting an object into it. In my experience, the former is more traumatic for the body.

BARBARA: And how are the results?

MIRHA-SOLEIL: I ended up with implants that are very hard. My left one is not too bad; I can live with it. But the right one is completely encapsulated which means it has developed a thick layer of scar tissue all around the implant. It also sits too high in relation to my left one. My nipple is almost under the breast. I felt there was something really wrong with my right breast soon after the surgery. The top of the breast was not only too high, but also puffy and too soft. I could feel the entire implant through my skin. It felt as if there was no breast tissue at all between the implant and the epidermis. I also lost all sensation in most of my right breast. It is now six months after the surgery and I still can't feel a thing in that area. I'm wondering if something happened during the surgery and they scraped away all my connective tissue and the nerve endings from that part of my breast.

I spoke to the surgeon several times after the surgery about my right breast being too high and about it feeling dead. He said sensation would return to normal at some point. I went back to see him a few weeks ago, five months after the surgery. My right breast had gotten really bad, it was so hard and looked quite deformed. His answers to my questions were all "yes" or "no." I was in his examining room for about one minute and thirty seconds, and he obviously wanted me out of there, and fast. He said he wanted to get me back in hospital to remove the scar tissue. He wants to do something called an open capsuloctomy. But he is insisting on also operating on my left one. He says that if he removes the scar tissue from the right one, then I will then find the left one too hard in comparison. I didn't want him to touch my perfectly fine left breast. I was too scared that the same thing that happened to my right breast would happen to my left one. But seeing another surgeon is like playing Russian roulette, so I chose to go ahead with him and to have him operate on both breasts. The surgery is scheduled for the first week of December 2000.

BARBARA: Is it physically painful?

MIRHA-SOLEIL: It's not painful, but uncomfortable, and not pretty! During all these years I have met and worked with numerous transsexual women who had all kinds of problems with their breast implants. I've also seen all kinds of results, both good and bad, from breast augmentations. Before the surgery, I formed for myself an image of the worst breasts that I could possibly get. And they're exactly what I got: breasts that are too high, hard, unnatural looking, dead and encapsulated. They don't look too bad when I have a bra and clothes on, but when I'm naked, they look like two horrendous balloons, one of which is deformed, stuck on my chest. However, I'm not too affected by them in my personal or professional life. As I explained earlier, my clients are very appreciative of various breast shapes and my boyfriend is very sweet and accepting, only I can't look at them in the mirror without thinking how awful they look, especially from the side. They are the breasts I had nightmares about prior to surgery. What's interesting though, is that now that I have these nightmarish breasts, I have learned to live with them. So I actually don't regret having had the surgery.

BARBARA: You don't regret it?

MIRHA-SOLEIL: Absolutely not. If somebody had told me that this is what I was going to get, I wouldn't have done it. But I don't regret it now because I like the way my breasts look with clothes on, my clients like them, and my boyfriend is not freaked out by them. The only thing that has changed is my willingness to show my naked body spontaneously in my art. I do performance art and experimental videos that often involve nudity, including mine. And while straight men are quite sweet about my screwed-up breasts, I don't expect the same sensitivity from artsy-fartsy crowds. I don't find artists to be particularly sensitive people in general, so I will be very careful in the future about using my naked breasts in my artwork. Nor am I comfortable showing my breasts to non-transsexual queer crowds. I recently had an invitation forwarded to me by a few non-transsexual friends about an upcoming "polymorphous" queer sex party. Even though these friends are nice people and they would make me feel comfortable being there, I can't imagine myself walking around as a woman with my dick and my deformed breasts in a primarily, perhaps exclusively, non-transsexual orgy! In a group of transsexual and transgendered people — yes, anytime. But I don't need non-transsexual dykes or fags checking out my tits to see how cement-like they feel. If you take my tits and put them in the mouth or hands of most genetic lesbians, even the sweetest and most sensitive ones, they will think, These tits are fucking hard! Now, give my tits to most transsexual men, transsexual women, or non-transsexual straight men who are used to sleeping with transsexual women, and because they have different standards, they'll just go, Yeah, nice tits.

That is a really strange feeling for me now, not being comfortable taking off my clothes in public spaces. I'm sort of back to stage one when I had "freakish" breasts as a child and teenager. I have little whining and crying sessions in my boyfriend's arms here and there about them, but it's not going to emotionally crush me. Over the years I have developed an ability to live with a body that doesn't fit the norm, a body that is somehow freakish, even repulsive to a lot of people. So a crooked tit is not going to make me break down.

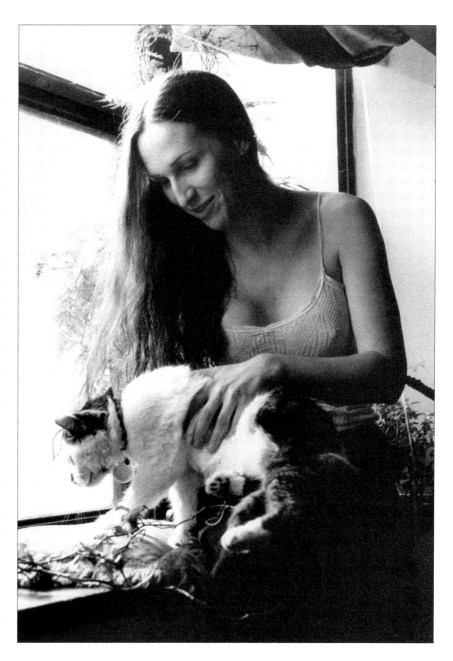

BARBARA: A lot of people say, "I'm going to make this choice so that my body better represents who I really feel I am inside." I hear you saying something a little different: that there is a comfort or strength that already exists in yourself, and that your body is the way it is.

MIRHA-SOLEIL: People always think that we change our bodies because we hate our bodies. I liked my breasts before my mastectomy, but I just couldn't go where I wanted to go with them. I even went through a mourning process that went with getting rid of my breasts, because I was emotionally attached to them. I had developed a relationship with them. I had struggled to accept them over the years. And, even more importantly, I wouldn't have been the same person if I hadn't had them. The same thing was true for the augmentation. I liked my small breasts, but I wanted to look like I had the breasts of a thirty year old woman.

BARBARA: Have you found that some people have made assumptions about why you made the decision to have breast surgery? That it somehow must have been imposed on you?

MIRHA-SOLEIL: Big topic! There's a lot of pressure coming from feminists to resist getting involved with cosmetic surgery, especially involving breast implants. I was so offended when, in the mid-nineties, I watched Gloria Steinem on television put down women who'd gotten cosmetic surgeries. She went into a big blah, blah, blah about how cosmetic surgery was all about mutilating our bodies in order to live up to patriarchal standards of beauty. I looked at this woman and thought, How arrogant! How dare she fucking judge! She looks stunning and is in her fifties. I don't think she has any clue what it's like to deal with real body issues. How condescending, demeaning it is to say that women choosing to get involved with cosmetic surgery are only doing so because of the pressure to live up to misogynistic standards of beauty. It is denying us any wisdom and agency in the decisions we make about our bodies and lives.

BARBARA: How has your feminist perspective informed your choices?

MIRHA-SOLEIL: I can't answer that question without also speaking about the anti-transsexual discourse that has been propagated by feminists since the seventies, a discourse that is now recycled by some transgendered

people, people who are excited about fucking up gender but not interested in radically changing their sex. Their analysis goes this way: If we weren't living in a binary gender system, we wouldn't have these counter-revolutionary transsexuals who mutilate their bodies in order to fit within narrow and oppressive sex/gender boxes. This was essentially the position articulated by anti-transsexual radical feminists such as Robin Morgan, Janice Raymond, Mary Daly, and also Gloria Steinem in the seventies.

This same frightening position is now being articulated by some transgendered activists and writers. I see many North American White Anglo transgendered activists who — when they are not too busy stealing indigenous spirituality and culture through their appropriation of the figure of the "berdache" and the concept of the "two spirit" — are getting involved with recycling backwards and reactionary seventies feminist, anti-transsexual discourses. And these people are even more dangerous because they appear to speak from the first person. So I see the attack on women who choose cosmetic surgery as coming from this same reductive, feminist discourse and political agenda, which proclaims that, if we weren't living in a patriarchal system, women wouldn't mutilate their flesh in order to live up to oppressive, patriarchal notions of female beauty.

So where do I stand in all of that? I think that even if we were living in this utopian "multi-gendered," perfect feminist culture on another planet 20,000 years from now, there would still be people who for all kinds of reasons would be driven to change their bodies and their sex. There can be something appealing, powerful and spiritual involved in body and sex changing, something that is stronger and wiser than just buying into society's stereotypes of what women and men should look like. For many of us, body- and sex-changing is an experience driven by a force that comes

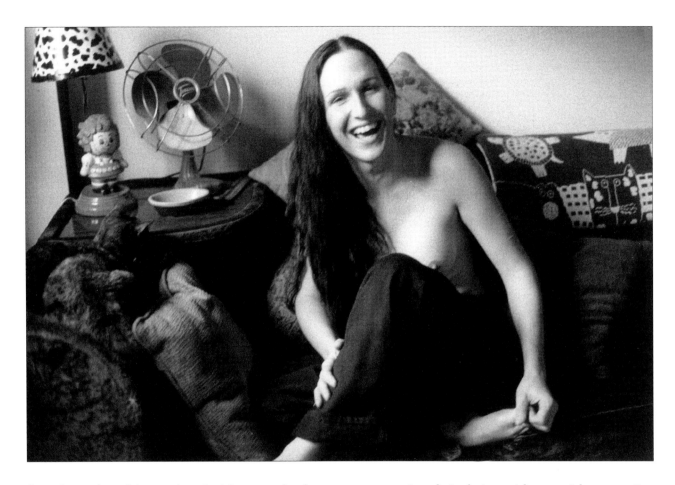

from beyond. Making such a decision can also be a form of political resistance to a judgemental and reductive feminist and transgender agenda. My plan for getting a vaginoplasty, for example, is a little bit in response to anti-transsexual feminist and transgender discourses. It is my way of saying, "Go to hell with your bullshit! I will show you that this little piece of skin I have between my legs is not immutable — that it is mine, that it doesn't determine my destiny, and that I will transform it as I see fit."

BARBARA: What do you recommend to people who are contemplating breast surgeries in terms of how they can negotiate their choices with potential surgeons?

MIRHA-SOLEIL: I think that any recommendation or suggestion — there were lots made to me — is useless as long as the power imbalance between surgeons and their clients remains. Suggestions are futile as long as we are desperate for a particular service that only certain surgeons can perform and then only if they are willing to do so.

So many people want cosmetic surgeries that clients are lining up months in advance for their appointments. If you won't comply with the surgeons' every wish, with their ideas of what you should get, or if you're too difficult a client, they will simply refuse to deal with you. They know they have another client anxiously waiting for an appointment to see them, ready to throw their money at them. The surgeons can pick and choose.

I'm a good example of someone who's informed about these issues, who knows what questions to ask, I'm someone who's grounded, able to stand up for herself — but I still didn't do too well at all because I didn't end up with what I wanted. I rarely find anybody who is completely satisfied with their nose job, or their lip job, or their boob job; the power imbalance that exists between surgeons and their patients is one factor that contributes to this level of dissatisfaction amongst cosmetic surgery clients. At this point it is very hard for me to completely assess my situation. I'm a little bit in limbo as I wait for the upcoming repair surgery to remove my scar tissue. I am quite scared of the potential results, but that won't stop me from going head on into it.

I have had a very complicated relationship with my breasts since I was very young, and this third breast surgery will not be the last breast surgery I get. I'm already thinking about getting bigger implants in two years. There are also some experiments going on in the United States with soya oil–filled implants and, as a vegan, this is something I find absolutely glamorous! I would love to be able to go around to social events and tell people I have soya tits! I would be so totally chic and sexy!

AFTERWORD

A few days before my boob repair job, I asked my surgeon about the chances of scar encapsulation reoccurring. He said there was a 30 percent chance of it happening again. Not too bad, I thought. "But if I were in that not-so-lucky 30 percent, what would I do?" He said in that case he'd have to remove the implants and try putting them under the muscles.

I was back in hospital in early December 2000. My surgeon was in a particularly good mood that day. He smiled and joked around a lot, which made me feel comfy and confident. Someone told me he had just had a kid.

I was lying down on my gurney, waiting in the hall by the operating room, when a man approached me and introduced himself as my anaesthesiologist. He was the sweetest knockout! He caressed my left arm and said, "I'll take care of you." I felt like I was sliding through some angel's fingers.

Things weren't so paradisiacal once I was in the operating room. My angelic anaesthesiologist asked a male paramedic in training to hook me up to the intravenous. I assumed that the IV was to give me some sugar because of my hypoglycaemia. I don't know if it was shock at meeting a transsexual or a French chick, or if it was that he saw that I had a nipple running up to my neck, but the poor paramedic became extremely nervous and started to shake. He struggled for about fifteen minutes before he was able to plug me in. He apologized for his clumsiness. I told him not to worry, just to make sure he was in my vein and not my bone.

I started to feel numb from the tip of my toes to the top of my head. I faded away slowly with an intense feeling of itchiness raging through my entire body. I realized they were putting me under intravenously instead of with a mask. I did not like that feeling; it lasted about a minute before I lost consciousness.

I woke up feeling extremely nauseous and sick because of the anaesthesia. My chest after this "open capsuloctomy" felt very similar to how my chest felt after my first breast surgery. I was in much more pain than I had been for the augmentation. I was also bleeding a lot, so I had tubes sticking out of the incisions to drain the blood for almost a week and a half.

During the first month after the surgery, my breasts appeared amazingly soft and natural but disappointingly small. Almost one-third of their former size had been scar tissue, which I'd grown used to and was now gone. Sniff! But as weeks went by, they started to grow bigger and harder and higher and weirder again. I am now nine months down the road, and they are both completely encapsulated again.

My right breast is a mess: the nipple is still running away under my arm; the implant is still too high; I still can't feel most of my breast, including the entire nipple; and, as a bonus, the scar is gruesome. It seems as if the skin of my right breast couldn't handle an incision twice in the same spot. It is puffed up, red and purple, and has developed bad keloid. None of it is really painful, but the whole breast feels extremely uncomfortable — depending on the weather!

I have since figured out on my own why my right breast is too high. The pocket the surgeon created for the implant is overly extended at the top of the breast, and my implant moves up into that empty space. I need to consult with another plastic surgeon to see if there's a way to tie that part of the skin back down onto the muscle. Doing that would put the nipple back in the middle of the breast.

I am taking a break for now to let my body rest, and I hope to be able to go back into surgery next year. I would like to change the implants from 300 cc to 400 cc and have them put under the muscle.

People are wondering if I'm bitter about my breasts not turning out to be top-notch. I am not because I am able to stand back and get some perspective. The outcome hasn't jeopardized my job, it hasn't hurt my relationship with my partner one bit, and it hasn't affected my physical or mental health. I am alive and able to make fun of it all.

And frankly, there are worse problems and tragedies all around us and in the world than a pair of tits gone haywire!

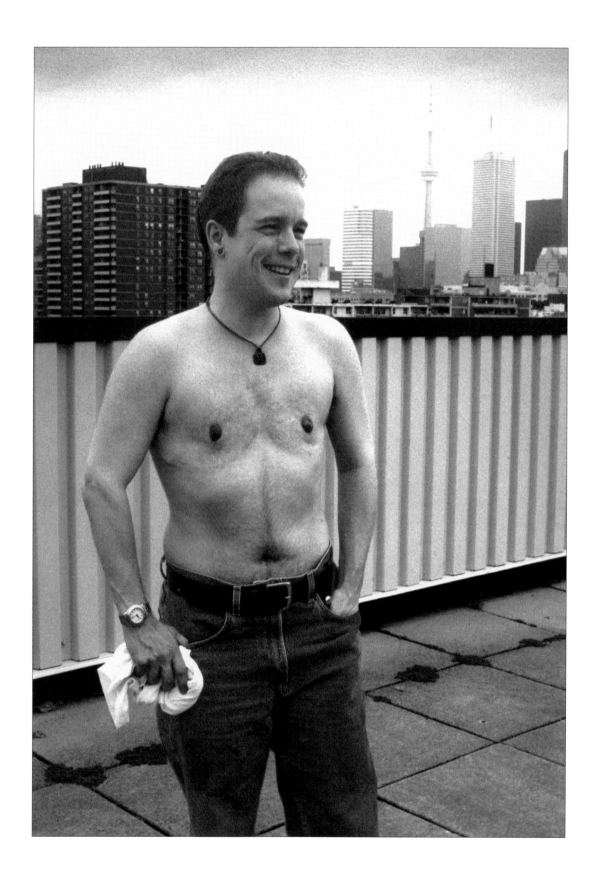

JAMES BROWN
The Person That I Am Now

A transsexual male in his late thirties, James Brown has had two surgeries: a breast reduction followed by a chest reconstruction surgery. In early adolescence, James felt himself to be male although he was biologically designated as female. Until he saw the show "The Wrong Body" on television, James wasn't fully able to identify his feelings, nor was he aware of what possibilities existed for him. Watching the documentary spurred James's actions toward surgery and transitioning at the age of thirty-three. James participated in a gender identity program through the mental health system, and thus was able to have his second surgery at a clinic specifically designed to perform transsexual surgeries.

James is a registered massage therapist and facilitates the FTM (female to male) Transition Support Group at the 519 Church Street Community Centre. He is interviewed by My Breasts, My Choice *editor Barbara Brown.*

JAMES: I should start by saying why it is that I want to be a part of this project. I have a story, and I'm tired of the feelings it brings up every time I talk about it. It is really stressful. If I could get the story out, it would be somewhere else. Then I could say, "Look at the installation. Get the book. Don't talk to me." I want to get the story out as one compact unit.

BARBARA: Just start your story at the beginning, although it must feel a little odd to think there's a formal beginning.

JAMES: I guess puberty is technically the beginning of the story for breasts. Before Grade Three, I used to go topless all the time. The neighbours complained because they thought it was inappropriate for little girls to go topless. My mother said, "Why are you complaining? She doesn't have anything there to notice." I wasn't aware of my chest for the most part. Then came puberty, when most girls would have to start wearing a bra. I was oblivious to the need until people at school told me I should be wearing one.

When I was twelve or thirteen years old, I began to bind my breasts for the first time ... I had pretty noticeable breasts by then, so I started binding because leather ties were in, and mine wouldn't hang properly, so I got a tensor bandage and bound my breasts. I thought, Wow, that looks really cool. It's really uncomfortable, but it looks great.

As far back as I can remember, I had questions about my gender. In 1979, when I was fourteen, I asked a boyfriend, "If I had a sex change, would you still date me?" Somehow I knew that transsexuals existed and that people could have sex changes. Later I asked my girlfriends the same thing.

Then — in the early eighties — a lot of women were not wearing bras out of political opposition to the fact that we were supposed to. I participated in that, but at the time I was an alcoholic. Because I was drunk a lot, I wasn't as aware when people stared at my chest.

I was really uncomfortable with having breasts. I didn't want lovers touching them. Most people I dated were horrified when I said I wanted to have them removed. Some even told me that no surgeon would ever do that for me, and they encouraged me to forget about it. Then I saw the show "The Wrong Body" on television. I realized that even though I was in my thirties, I could still do something about the way I felt about my body. Within two weeks of seeing that show, I was at a gender identity disorder clinic filling out the forms and getting into the program. This was the beginning of my transition from female-to-male.

I decided to start going to the transition support group at the 519 Church Street Community Centre in January 1997 to meet other transsexual people. I started hormones in March of that year. In June, I had my first appointment with the gender identity disorder [GID] clinic.

When I first went to see an endocrinologist for the hormones in March, he recommended a reduction mammoplasty before doing a real-life test. He felt there was no way I was going to "pass" (I hate that term) as a guy with 44DD breasts. I agreed with him. I wanted to start the real-life test right away, so I began phoning surgeons.

I had heard that some surgeons would do a complete chest reconstruction but would write it down as a breast reduction so that it could be covered by the Ontario Health Insurance Plan [OHIP]. However, it was almost impossible to find one who would do this for me. Either the surgeons wouldn't do it at all, or they had to have approval from a recognized gender identity disorder clinic. I finally decided to go with a Toronto surgeon. He offered to perform the chest reconstructive surgery for $5,000, but I couldn't afford that much. He suggested a reduction mammoplasty [breast reduction] and I asked how small he could make them. "An A," he said. OHIP would pay for a

reduction so I said, "Okay, let's do it."

I had surgery on July 29, 1997, and then started school in September, six months after starting on testosterone. In the gender identity disorder clinic's program everyone is expected to do a real-life test for at least one year before starting hormones, and then do a second year on hormones before surgery. Because I went on hormones prior to starting the program, I was permitted to continue them even though the clinic staff could have made it more difficult for me to get in because I wasn't doing it their way.

BARBARA: What is the real-life test?

JAMES: The real-life test requires that you be a full-time student, a full-time volunteer, or be employed for twelve consecutive months while living in your new gender. I went to university.

After the surgery and the hormones had begun to take effect, I looked a lot younger than thirty-three. People didn't believe me when I told them how old I was, so I stopped telling them. I had just been getting used to the fact that I was over thirty and that people were treating me like an adult. It was strange then to suddenly be a guy and look seventeen — people were treating me like a kid. They'd make comments or change their tone of voice when they spoke to me. Sometimes they just ignored me. I had to relax and not worry about it. During the following two years my body changed again from being on the hormones and I aged ten years! And then I aged another ten due to hair loss, which can be a side-effect of testosterone replacement therapy.

BARBARA: How old are you now?

JAMES: I'm thirty-seven. After I had been in the gender identity disorder clinic's program for one and a half years, OHIP cut the funding — or rather, the provincial government cut the funding to OHIP for transsexual surgeries, claiming they were elective and not medically necessary.

I wasn't sure what to do. I talked to a credit union manager who was very supportive and gave me a line of credit even though I had no collateral. That line of credit allowed me to have the final top surgery in May 2000. For this operation, I chose to go to a clinic in Montreal that specializes in transsexual surgeries and is known to have the top surgeons in this field in Canada. The surgeon contoured my chest to appear male and removed most of the thick scar tissue left behind from the previous chest surgery. I also feel really lucky, because I know people who have had to have nipple grafts. At least my surgery didn't involve having to cut my nipples off, move them and sew them back on. After the surgery, you have to bind your chest for six weeks to reduce the swelling.

Sometimes it kills me to listen to people who have had their top surgery complain during their first six months of transition, "Ooh, I had to bind for seven months before surgery." I had to bind for three years after the first surgery. I'm really glad it's done.

I want to go back and talk about the two surgeries in more detail now. The first surgery, the breast reduction, which occurred in a Scarborough hospital, was a bit of a disaster. A lot of things went wrong. Two weeks before the surgery, I did something to my neck and I ended up with pain shooting down my arm. Because you're not supposed to take certain medications, including aspirin, prior to surgery, I couldn't do anything about it. It was so painful.

Then a friend, who is also FTM [female to male], was going to take me to the hospital, and he locked his keys in the car. I ended up taking a taxi, and he met me there later. After the surgery — it was day surgery in a hospital — his car broke down on the highway and the passenger side door was right up against the guard-rail and could not be opened. I ended up having

to crawl out of the window. I had to wait on the side of the road for a taxi just hours after my surgery!

At home, I didn't have anyone to look after me. One friend did stay over the first night, but she is grumpy and doesn't like sick people very much. That wasn't helpful for me. Then I got an infection because I hadn't been given the proper after-care instructions by the surgeon. He had recommended using a six-inch tensor bandage and a tight sports bra on top to create pressure on the incisions and reduce swelling. It was difficult to put the sports bra on, though, because I had to pull it over my head, but I wasn't supposed to raise my arms after the surgery. I also had a hard time putting the tensor bandage on by myself. After the surgery I was using Tylenol 3 because I still had nerve pain down my arm, but that meant I couldn't feel if I was pulling on any of the stitches. I think all those things contributed to the infection and some of the scarring.

The last thing I had to deal with was that the skin on my chest did not come together properly. For the breast reduction surgery they cut up the centre of the breast to the nipple and then under the breast, remove the breast tissue, and then pull the skin together. The patch at the bottom in the centre where the skin is supposed to fit together didn't come together on me. It healed into a big lump of scar tissue. Because the surgeon cut the pedicle [stalk of nerves and blood supply] of my left nipple, it turned completely black, and I didn't know if I was going to get to keep it or not.

BARBARA: What happened?

JAMES: The black stuff formed a scab on my nipple and eventually fell off. The scar tissue is still there. I didn't lose the actual nipple, but I did lose sensation in it. Sensation in the right nipple remained, though, as the surgeon did not cut the pedicle on the right side. Oddly, since the second surgery, some of the sensation in my left nipple has returned, but now I've lost sensation in my right nipple.

Once I had arranged for the second operation, the chest reconstruction, I decided that I would take all kinds of vitamins before and after the surgery. My chiropractor gave me a list of the right ones. I took zinc, vitamin C, B6, and colostrum. After surgery I used MSM cream for tissue repair and tea-tree oil to dry up a small infection I had. The tea-tree oil was very effective.

BARBARA: Did you have a health-care professional overseeing this self-treatment?

JAMES: No; it was too expensive. I studied nutrition at school so I decided to use the information in my nutritional healing book instead. I was really excited about the second surgery. I knew about it six months beforehand, in part because the funding cuts meant I'd had to make the special arrangements to pay for it.

BARBARA: How much did this surgery cost?

JAMES: About $4,700. The Montreal clinic specializes in transsexual surgeries, including FTM chest reconstructive surgery, metoidioplasty, and phalloplasty. The cost covered a five-day stay at the residence, including all meals, nursing care and limo service between the residence and the train station or airport.

The clinic had a few general requirements. First, they required that candidates have a recommendation from a psychiatrist, which I had. I was lucky, because in 1997, before going into the GID clinic's program, I had seen a psychiatrist recommended by my family doctor. I had needed to get a letter of approval for the chest reconstructive surgery, just in case the GID clinic required me to wait too long. I still had that letter. The psychiatrist had stopped practising, but when I sent the letter to Montreal in November 1999, the clinic accepted it. They also required anyone having chest

reconstructive surgery to have been on hormones for at least a year. This gives the chest muscles time to develop a bit and makes it easier for the surgeon to reconstruct following the outline of the new muscle. I was fine because I had been on testosterone for three years by the time I had surgery. They also wanted me to be near normal body weight. After the first surgery, I had weighed 178 pounds. I started losing weight in November 1999 and I was down to 150 pounds when I had the second surgery. I've continued to lose weight and have lost a total of forty-five pounds. I think being thinner helps in terms of "passing" for FTMs.

I had the second surgery in May 2000. I arrived in Montreal by train, and the clinic's limo driver was there to pick me up. I was driven to the residence, which was staffed around the clock by nurses. The doctor met with me on the first day and we discussed what was going to happen. In addition to the chest surgery, I was able to arrange for liposuction in the area under my arms. The next day, the surgeon arrived at the residence to drive me and the other guy having surgery that day to the clinic! It was cool sitting and talking with the surgeon in his car on the way there. At the clinic, after being assigned a room, I was introduced to the anaesthesiologist.

The surgeon also drove me back to the residence after the surgery. I talked with other people at the residence who had had the same surgery. Some had had it a couple of days before, and some were there for surgical revisions. The doctor came and checked on me the next day, and I saw him often during the five days I stayed at the residence following the surgery.

While I was at the residence, the nurses showed me how to look after my chest and the incisions. During the surgery, the doctor had inserted two tubes into my skin that looked like flattened, perforated straws. The straws wrapped around either side of my chest and were there to reduce the swelling. I also had a small opening in the skin under each arm for a tube that was connected to a bulb. I had to maintain a certain amount of pressure on the bulb to help the fluid drain. I'd empty the bulb once or twice a day. It was wild. I'd sit up and hear gurgling noises coming from my chest! It was kind of gross. The drains were taken out on the last day before I went home.

I had one person stay the first night I was home but that was all. Because I'd had the five days of recovery time at the clinic, I was fine on my own. This time my healing went a lot better.

I am a firm believer in socialized medicare, but after those two experiences, I thought, If I could afford it, I'd go with private health care all the way. I really enjoyed the kind of interaction I had with the doctors and staff. I thought all the care and attention I received from people there was great.

BARBARA: What were the differences you noticed between the two surgical experiences?

JAMES: For the first surgery, the surgeon seemed very distant with me. We had an initial consultation and he talked about what he was going to do, but I didn't see him in the hospital at all before the surgery, although I'd wanted to. In the hospital the administrative personnel took all my stuff away from me (including my glasses) and left me in a huge room with a ton of people all waiting for surgery. I was wheeled into the operating room and the surgeon

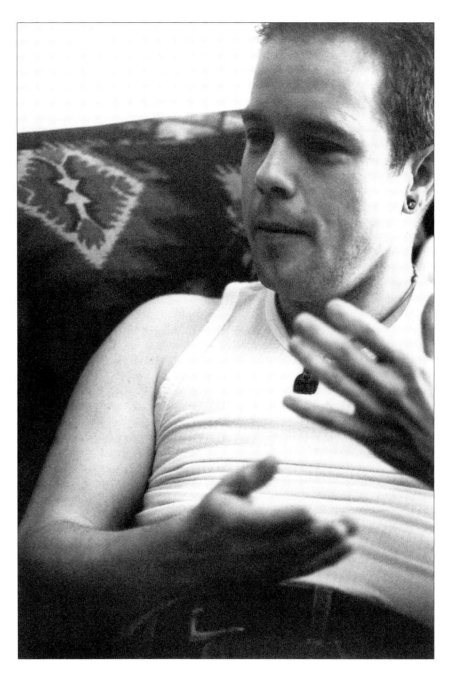

drew on my chest where he was going to cut. I again asked him to try to make my chest as flat as possible. I was lucky to even have five seconds of interaction with him before they put me out.

I felt worried. *Oh, my god. What is he going to do?*

I really hope he knows what it is that I want. But basically, it was up to him. I wasn't even guaranteed that he would be the one to sew me back up, as we were in a teaching hospital. I woke up in another big room on a gurney with a different bunch of people lying on their gurneys; fortunately, someone came to check on me because I was having trouble breathing.

The biggest difference between the surgeries was that at the Montreal clinic, a private clinic, I felt like a person, whereas at the Scarborough hospital, a public institution, I felt like just another patient.

BARBARA: What about activities after the reconstructive surgery? What were you able to do?

JAMES: Three days later I went to a film festival party. I felt some pulling around the incision, but overall, everything was fine. I didn't lift things or raise my hands over my head. I had the most pain where I'd had the liposuction under my arms. Three weeks after the surgery this area was still really painful if I brushed my skin against anything or wore a backpack.

BARBARA: Did they explain the process of liposuction?

JAMES: I don't know what approach they used, but the area is still numb. The next surgery I have to think about is a hysterectomy, which I am not looking forward to. I have heard that Kitchener is the place to go, because there's a gynaecologist there who does good work, and it's not day surgery. In Toronto it would be. It seems weird to leave the city to have surgery.

BARBARA: Is the hysterectomy related to your transition?

JAMES: It's medically recommended to have a hysterectomy before four years on testosterone injections, because there is a risk of developing cervical and ovarian cancer. I've been on it for four and a half years now. The hysterectomy would also allow me to reduce my hormone dosage, which would be better for my liver.

Reactions to my surgery have been scary! My best friend, who thought about transitioning at one point, has said a variety of things to me over the past four years. In the beginning what she said was hard to hear. She said things like, "I wouldn't want to be a freak." I said, "Are you saying that I'm a freak?" She said, "No, no. For me, *I* would feel like a freak." I thought, It doesn't matter if you rephrase that, it still feels like you're telling me that that's how you see me.

She thinks my chest looks okay now. She can't believe how much the scars have faded. Her breasts are really large, and she hates the physical pain they cause her. She thought about having reduction surgery, but she doesn't want the scars. For me, the scars suck, but compared to what I was living with, it's not really worse.

BARBARA: How was your life pre-transition and before your two surgeries?

JAMES: Oh, don't make me go there! How was it before? I just hated it. I didn't like going outside. I didn't like that everywhere I went people stared at my chest and even if I didn't notice that people were staring, others I was with would say, "That guy is staring at your chest." I got to a point where I would no longer be aware of my surroundings because I couldn't deal with the constant harassment from men. I couldn't go three blocks from my house without somebody yelling or saying something harassing to me on the street.

Now I go out and no one says anything to me except maybe to ask me for change or a cigarette. Maybe I was giving off that whole victim thing, who knows? But then you'd think I'd stil be giving it off.

BARBARA: I think those kinds of things don't come at us just because we're putting something out. We live in a cultural context.

JAMES: Right, but if that's the case, it should happen to everyone. My best friend is at least as big as I was, and no one ever says a word to her. Ever. So I don't know. She said, "It's because you're blond." I talked to other blond people. It wasn't that. I don't know what it was.

BARBARA: How did you feel about your breasts at that time?

JAMES: I just wanted to get rid of them. At that point, even if it meant being horribly scarred, it would have been worth it to me. That's a terrible way to think, because of course after it's over it would matter if I were horribly scarred. But I felt desperate and I even started to have weird thoughts of doing it myself. I thought, Get these tumours off my chest.

I've heard people say, and I agree, that it doesn't seem right that women can go and get implants to make their breasts larger than anatomically possible, whereas, if we want to have them removed, we have to go for a psychiatric assessment. It's bizarre.

BARBARA: It's not seen as anything wrong if you want them a little smaller.

JAMES: No one sees a reduction as wrong if it is to relieve back pain. If someone wants the surgery for any other reason, though, then that's viewed as weird.

BARBARA: What other kinds of things have people said to you?

JAMES: I hate this one — everyone always says to me, "I guess you're going to have to build up your chest now!" I want to say to them, "I guess you're going to have to lose some weight." I don't get it. I have my breasts removed and now I have to become a body-builder? It is totally not cool for them to say that to me.

The other day my friend and I were in a change room. Since I've lost weight, I've noticed that my rib cage sticks out. My best friend said, "Oh, that's really gross." I suppose it *is* kind of weird; other guys I've seen don't usually have ribcages that stick out. I guess they are built differently on top. I *would* like to work out, but not to make them shut up — just because it's something I want to do.

BARBARA: Do you think that other people believe they have the right to speak out about your body because of the choices you've made along the way? Do you think it's a cultural thing? Where do you think these people's comments come from?

JAMES: I think I have rude friends! Most of them are exes of mine, so they feel they have licence. One friend came over and said, "You have really girlie legs." I don't know what that's all about. It's as if people split me into two — the person that I was before transition and the person that I am now — as if we were actually different individuals, not just two parts of me.

BARBARA: How do you experience yourself?

JAMES: I'm still me. I don't split myself. I haven't rewritten my past. Sometimes I'll be talking about being a teenager and say, "my boyfriend." It sounds as if I was gay at thirteen, a boy with a boyfriend, not a female with a guy. Recently it isn't as big a deal as it once was that people think I'm gay because I don't care anymore. I've joined a gay men's chorus, and I'm not as hard on myself about who I'm attracted to. When I first came out as trans it was a big deal. I only knew one other FTM, and for him being a man was about being butch and masculine, which I just am not.

My family has reacted in different ways. My aunt has had a really hard time with my transition. She says I still look the same, which my uncle thinks is hysterical. My mother's been really cool though — she calls me James and uses the right pronouns. She introduces me as her son and is really proud of me.

My sister, however, uninvited me to Christmas, once I decided to transition, and I haven't seen her or her kids for four and a half years. My mother hasn't been able to see the kids either for a couple of years. That's hard. My sister thinks my transitioning would be hard on them, and doesn't trust that my mother would keep me from seeing them. When my aunt invites the family over for holiday meals, my mother says if I am not invited, she won't go either. I think that cutting my sister's kids off from their grandmother and me is hard on them too.

BARBARA: Your dad?

JAMES: My dad died when I was thirteen.

The big thing that was hard for me in my previous relationships was that people needed to see me as "femme." I pulled it off so that I could get what I wanted in terms of being with the people I was attracted to and finding sexual satisfaction.

BARBARA: You got what you wanted because you were femme?

JAMES: If I had insisted that everyone see me as male back then, with the way I looked, I probably would never have been able to date anyone. They were attracted to what they saw on the outside. Of course, they were disappointed when they started dating me and realized the inside didn't match the outside. It bugged me that the first thing people were drawn to were my breasts. That was the one thing that I didn't want people to be attracted to, but it was consistent. They'd deny that my breasts were the lure, but if I wore a fancy bra, their eyes would light up.

I had to make some difficult decisions before transitioning: one, I had to be ready to accept that I might lose my voice, from the effects of testosterone, and I'm a singer. And two, I needed to be okay with the fact that I might never date again, because people might be freaked out that what they saw on the outside didn't match what was underneath my clothing. I figured that after transition I would never be with anyone ever again. I worried that the way they would see me would make me feel creepy about myself. I wondered if people would treat me like a woman, even though I'm not. I decided that even if I had to give up relationships and even if I had to give up my voice, being a guy was more important. Life prior to transition was so horrendous that I couldn't stand it anymore. Fortunately, I have gotten my voice back to some degree, although it's not as good as before, and I'm dating someone now.

I went to a women's bathhouse a while back. It was the first time I'd been in a swimming pool since I transitioned. One woman asked me if I was a man. I didn't know how to answer the question, because the categories didn't fit. I just said, "Yeah, sort of." It bothered her that I was in the change room. I said, "That's fine. I'm getting my stuff and I'm leaving. See ya." Other than that, I had no problems there. It was really great. I didn't go for sex; I went for the whirlpool and the steam room, and just to relax.

BARBARA: You need to get out a little more!

JAMES: Where else would I go? I can't go to most swimming facilities, because I can't use the open showers without the bottom surgery. It was nice to have a place where I could just relax. Many years ago I went to the Michigan Womyn's Music Festival. I was a separatist lesbian at the time. It was nice to be away from men because I really didn't want them looking at me in a harassing, sexual way. When I was between seventeen and nineteen years old, I was in the armed forces. Guys would say to me, "You're just one of the guys," but they still didn't treat me as one sometimes.

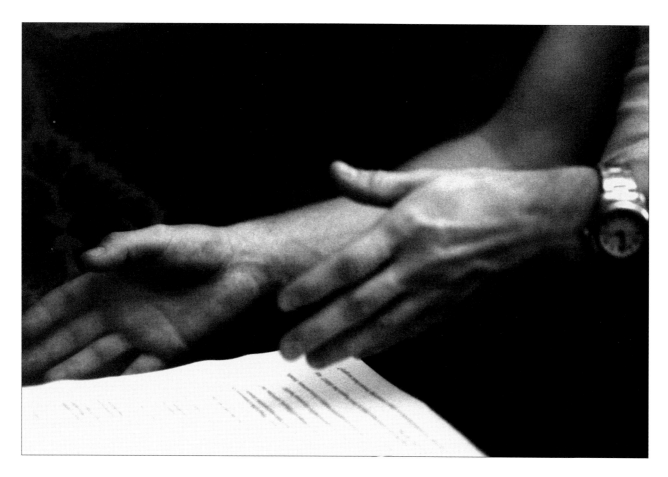

BARBARA: Have you completed the gender identity program?

JAMES: No, I haven't. This is the ridiculous part. At the end of the two years, they said, "You failed these courses at school, so that means you haven't been successful in the real-life test. Obviously it's not working for you."

I said, "It's the organic chemistry. I suck at organic chemistry and math." But they were insistent, and told me I had to do more time as a part of the real-life test. So I completed another term.

I then met with a doctor at the GID clinic in September 2000 for my final assessment. I didn't hear back from them until July 2001. Depending on who I spoke with, the doctor hadn't returned his calls or he had gone on vacation or they hadn't received his paperwork. And now the paperwork's been lost. I am scheduled to go back on September 17 for, hopefully, my last session.

Once I have approval, if I ever want lower surgery — if lower surgery improves or if there is funding, or if I move to another province where it is already funded, such as Alberta or BC — then I won't have to go through the whole psychiatric assessment and real-life test again. That's why I'm doing the program. Plus, I've put in so much time, and I want the documentation. Maybe I'll frame it! So many people start but drop out or decide that they don't want to have anything to do with it — or they can afford to decide that. The cost for lower surgery is minimum $10,000, plus any corrections over the years. That's a lot of money that I don't have.

UPDATE

Since the interview with Barbara, I have been back to the gender identity disorder clinic, and it looks like I will be getting their approval. Both the psychologist and the head psychiatrist were very pleased with my transition. Although I don't like the program, and think the criteria are archaic, I am still glad I went through it. I work in health care and also facilitate an FTM peer support group, so I understand both sides of the issue. Because of this work experience, I have been able to negotiate my way through their program in ways that some other TG/TS [transgendered/ transsexual] folks haven't been able to.

There are medical guidelines for the care of TG/TS people called the "Harry Benjamin International Gender Dysphoria Association [HBIGDA] Standards of Care for Gender Identity Disorders." The guideline for hormone administration is "a documented real life experience of at least three months prior to the administration of hormones" or, that the person should undergo "a period of psychotherapy of a duration specified by the mental health professional (usually three months) after an initial evaluation."

The gender identity disorder clinic program that I was in required me to live a full year in my new gender without hormones. I think that this time period is unrealistic, and I think that most, if not all, people in the program end up starting hormones with a family doctor before the year is over.

When I was in the program, I was asked, as others are, intimate questions about who I was dating and what my sexual orientation was. Luckily, I was dating a woman and said so. I was also dating another FTM, but I didn't volunteer this information because I had heard stories from other FTMs who dated men and shared the information with people at the clinic. When they did, they were told that homosexual attraction is unusual, and they would have to undergo psychiatric assessment and counselling before being approved for hormone treatment.

To me there seemed to be a bias toward heterosexuality. I believe the people making the assessments didn't take into account the psychological impact of people's histories, especially if there was abuse. They didn't clarify for themselves the difference between gender and sexual orientation and instead relied on outmoded stereotypes of what it means to be male or female. I was affected by these beliefs in the program, and have met and worked with many FTMs who were also affected by them.

I do think it's important to screen for mental illness and to test what people's ways for dealing with stress are, because transition is hard and stressful. I also understand the program's need for documentation, and for people to do a real-life test of some sort to make sure that people know that this is what they want. I just think that the GID clinic needs to consider that there are many variations of men and woman. Not all women wear dresses everyday and not all men wear suits and ties. Not all people are heterosexual. I think the GID clinic needs to embrace diversity a bit more.

I'm glad I went through the program, because it medically legitimizes my transsexuality. My family, especially my aunt, was better able to understand my decision to transition knowing that doctors were monitoring my progress. The fact that medical specialists thought I was transsexual meant more to my aunt than the fact that I did. I'm not happy about that, but it served a purpose at the time.

A lot of FTMs resent that the program medicalizes and pathologizes transsexuals. They don't like it being listed in the DSM [Diagnostic Statistical Manual]. I think, though, that if we want government funding for surgery, we benefit from being in the manual. For me, the result of completing the program is documentation that will allow me to obtain further SRS [sexual reassignment surgery], should I desire it. I still haven't written off the idea of phalloplasty, but at the moment I am pretty happy with what I have.

I am a registered massage therapist. While I was in school, I was one of the few people who felt uncomfortable receiving breast massage. After graduation I also had trouble with male clients coming on to me and asking for "extras." I worked in a couple of downtown hotel massage clinics and spas. When I decided to transition, I let my registration become inactive for almost three years. I've just recently reactivated my registration and I and hope to build up my practice around treating transsexual and transgender clients. I know from my own experience that transition can be a lonely time. I became quite touch-starved. Post-surgery, I worked on my own scars and showed other FTMs how to massage their scars to make them less noticeable. I think there is a real need in the TG/TS community for health-care practitioners who are accepting and knowledgeable of the gender transition process.

FINAL NOTE

I received my approval letter from the GID clinic in August 2002, almost five and a half years after starting their program. The letter gives me approval for metoidioplasty. This is good because it allows me the option of lower surgery in the future, should I desire it. Mostly, I just wanted some form of documentation that stated that I survived their program. An MTF friend of mine said, "The way I think of it is that it is nice to have undergone a psychiatric examination — and passed!" I agree.

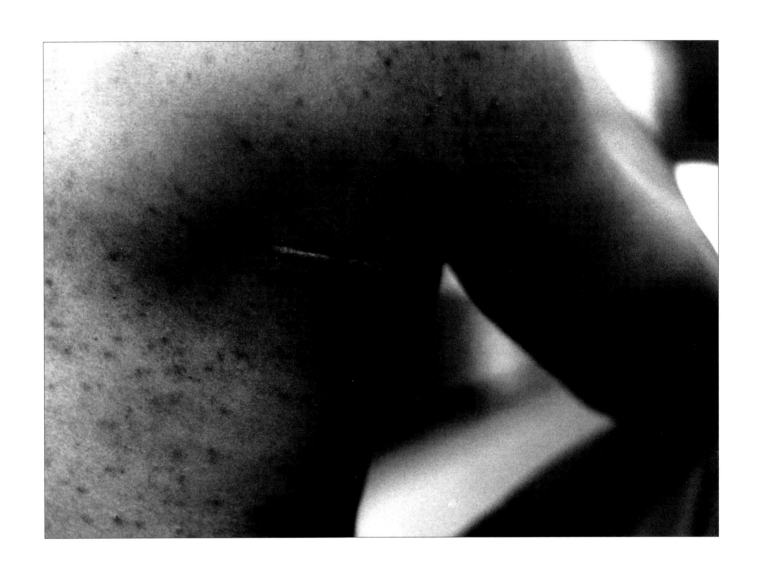

Kevin's Story
Living With What's Done

A gay man in his thirties, Kevin pursued corrective surgery for gynaecomastia (development of breast tissue in men). His gynaecomastia was related to use of liver medications, and may have been exacerbated by use of steroid-based nutritional supplements. Kevin tried weight loss and weight training to reduce the size of his chest, but was unsuccessful. His first surgery was performed by a surgeon who initially said he'd done "hundreds" of such operations. After the surgery, Kevin discovered the surgeon had only done three gynaecomastia corrective surgeries on men. And, in fact, the surgeon did not perform a reduction/excision procedure but rather did liposuction. The chemical injection from the liposuction and fatty tissue removal process left Kevin with severe burns and scars, many of them permanent. His chest size was not reduced significantly and one nipple became inverted. When Kevin pursued legal recourse, he discovered that this surgeon had other patients who had previously attempted to sue, all unsuccessfully. Kevin dropped the legal action and contacted a second — reputable — surgeon who performed the gynaecomastia correction. Kevin is pleased with the outcome, although he had to carry the costs for both surgeries, a serious economic strain.

Kevin has maintained complete anonymity in the project.

When I was a kid growing up, I never really had a flat, flat chest. I had fat on my chest, but never so much that I felt uncomfortable. I have never been very muscular either, but for the last fifteen years or so, I've worked out fairly regularly.

In 1995, I developed a serious liver condition that required medication. After I had taken it for two to three months, my chest started hurting. I was told the medication had upset my hormonal balance, which may have caused my breasts to start developing. Eventually the problem with my liver was solved; everything went back to normal. My breasts went back to their original size and my liver was as healthy as can be. After a year, I went off the medication.

Just shortly after my liver condition was diagnosed, I went through a rough period after a break-up. My liver condition had made me weak. When I had enough energy, I began working out a lot to build my self-esteem, doing the old I'm-so-desirable thing. Occasionally I took creatine, a strength-building supplement. I had been taking different protein supplements on and off since 1992. Later I would learn that the creatine may also have had something to do with my breasts developing.

About two years later, in 1997, I began noticing that my breasts were getting a little more pronounced, although not noticeably to others or enough to make me uncomfortable. I just thought, Oh, my pecs are getting quite developed. Later in that same year, however, they started getting pointy. I began to wear a tight tank top under my shirt to flatten my breasts and ultimately it got to where I also wore a t-shirt under my tank top. Then while attending a family gathering, my sister — you know how lovely siblings can be —

pointed out to everyone that I had breasts. I looked in the mirror and thought, Oh, my god, it's true. They're bigger than I thought. With that realization, I no longer felt comfortable going without my t-shirt and tank top. Later that year, I went to the tropics with my family, and I couldn't bring myself to expose my chest on the beach with my breasts looking like they did. I'm not saying that my sister put this idea into my head. I only know I couldn't stop thinking, They're breasts. They're pointing out.

I started doing some research. I learned from my doctor that the breast development was probably a side-effect of the medication I took for my liver flare up. When I first started taking the medication, side-effects involving a potential hormonal imbalance were mentioned, but I didn't pay much attention. My medical condition was so bad that I couldn't do anything but sleep. When I was told that the medication would help, if not correct, my liver problem, I didn't complain. I just took it. I didn't concern myself with possible side-effects. I also learned the breast tissue growth might have been influenced by the high-protein supplements I'd been taking. Sometimes when men have too much protein in their systems, it can disrupt their estrogen balance, causing breasts to grow.

No way existed, however, to absolutely nail down the source. I cut back on taking the protein supplement, creatine, and I continued to work out. I was uncomfortable taking my shirt off but still liked my body. I'm not blaming anybody for the breast tissue growing; I just didn't want to have it on my chest.

The physical and emotional discomfort and the necessity of having to wear a tight tank top and t-shirt continued from 1997 until 1998, until I realized that my breasts had gotten even bigger. Because of other issues in my life, I had stopped working out so often. Initially I had thought my breasts were my pectoral muscles that were getting too heavy, but I didn't have

the muscular arms and shoulders that might have made my breasts look like part of the whole body-building thing. Even though I wasn't working out as much, my breasts remained. I also began to think that maybe I was still dealing with the effects of the medication. I began to feel really sensitive about how I looked. If I went to the gym, I'd never shower there. Even if I stank, I wouldn't take my shirt off. I'd wait until I got home.

I got to a point where I wasn't interested in having sex with anybody I found extremely attractive and appealing. Instead I was having sex with people I didn't really care about, people I couldn't possibly be interested in emotionally. I wouldn't take my shirt off and let them see my chest. I'd say, "No, I want to keep this on." I didn't have any qualms about saying, "No, I'm not taking it off." If they started reaching for my chest, I'd move their hands. Eventually this became a chore. I was getting sick of doing it and I didn't want my life to continue this way. If I care about somebody, I definitely want to please him — I want to give him the maximum amount of pleasure. At this point, however, I could not put myself through having someone I cared for touch or see me.

By 1998 I had started thinking about corrective surgery. I decided, I'm not going to have sex with anybody until these things are off. I didn't want to risk anybody saying in the dark, "My god, what are these?" Guys want to feel pecs, they don't want to feel breasts. It became a major issue for me, and a source of serious depression.

When I found out how much the surgery would cost, I tried everything to come up with the money. Unfortunately though, things were really bad financially, and I realized I couldn't afford surgery. I was willing to ignore my rent for a few months to cover the cost of the surgery, but I wasn't even able to pay my rent because I was so financially stretched. So for three more years, my situation just kept getting worse. I lost a lot of my self-esteem. I didn't feel like going to the gym at all any more because I thought, What's the point? I discovered that working out actually made my breasts protrude even more and when I stopped working out, I lost chest muscle and ended up with droopy breasts. I stopped having sex entirely, and just kept hoping and praying for the day when I could afford to remove them.

I wanted to grow old gracefully, but I didn't want to grow old with breasts. I know that some men as they grow older start getting bigger, softer chests. I can accept this on some — older men and men who are overweight. But I looked like an adolescent girl. When I walked quickly, my breasts would bounce. They hurt, too. My chest was very sensitive to touch. I finally realized what women go through when they grow breasts.

I have a young spirit, and I feel I have a lot more living to do and a lot more fun to have. I'm also single and I'm looking for a partner. I'm not wealthy enough to buy myself a little toy-boy, and I wouldn't want that. I simply want to be comfortable with myself, and continue to do things that are right for me. I decided to have the surgery not to make myself happy, but to make myself less unhappy. If the change had been gradual, say over a period of ten years, I could have accepted it more easily than what I ended up having to deal with. I could say, Okay, I saw it coming. But this happened in less than three years — *boom!*

I don't want to be perfect. I've never wanted to be

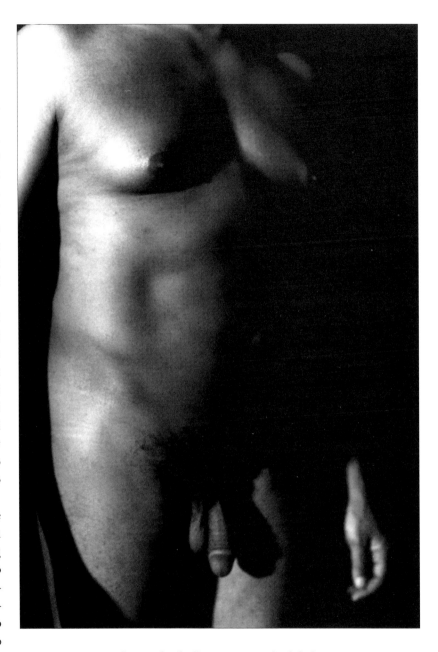

perfect. I think flaws are wonderful things in everybody, but this was something that made me feel miserable. I felt the need to do whatever I could about my breasts to make myself feel better. I didn't want to play the victim. I just felt, No, I can't live with this. Not now in my life, no. It just wasn't something I was willing to live with. I knew I wasn't doing this for anybody else. I decided to have the surgery because my body made me feel very, very uncomfortable. The surgery was going to give me a chance to be free again, free of having female breasts.

I began to research surgeons who do breast tissue removal. The doctor recommended by my physician was heavily booked. Each time I made an appointment, I thought I would have the money but then didn't, so I'd have to postpone. Every time that happened, it would be six months again before I could see him again — just for a consultation. When I finally got some money in my hands, I did some quick checking around and came across another clinic that could perform the reduction procedure right away. I booked with them so I wouldn't have to wait any longer. I thought about the procedure, It can't be that complicated. These people do this all the time. Let it be done, and let me be free of this baggage that I've been carrying around for such a long time.

My motivation to proceed with the surgery and my decision about the clinic had a lot to do with wanting to get involved with somebody, but not until I'd had the surgery. If I met someone I cared about, I'd say, I hope he doesn't get involved with anybody for the next six months. Let me just get myself back together, and then I'll ask him out. The way I looked at it was — and I wasn't beating up on myself by saying it — how could I expect anybody to go to bed with me while I had these breasts when *I* would never sleep with anybody who had them? It seems to me that males are very vain. As a man interested in men, I am very visually stimulated. And I wasn't going to put myself through the torture of rejection by someone I cared about. I've not been rejected by anybody up to now because I haven't given anybody the chance.

I had the surgery in July 2001. I had stopped working out so that my breast tissue wouldn't be as defined. Before the surgery I said to the surgeon, "You

need to remove the breast tissue, because I don't want these things to continue to grow." The surgeon said, "The liposuction will take care of that." But I said, "No, you need to cut it out."

In our consultation right before the surgery, when he was drawing lines on my chest, I asked, "Why aren't you making the incision at the nipples?" He said, "It's better to do the surgery from the armpit so there's no scarring." I asked, "Can you cut out the breast tissue from the armpit?" And he said, "Yes, we can. We'll take care of that."

During the weeks after the surgery, when I was in so much physical pain, I discovered that he had simply removed my fat tissue with liposuction. I felt a lot of emotional pain in realizing that he had not actually removed my breast tissue.

After the surgery, I wore what looked like a girdle around my chest. I was supposed to wear the girdle for two weeks. Two days after the surgery I went in to get things checked out because my chest was painful as hell and I had a lot of bruising. The surgeon said the pain was from fluid in one breast that could be removed after the girdle came off. When the two weeks were up, I went back to see him, and he said, "No, there's still a lot of swelling. You'll have to wear it for another week." I went to see him a week after that, only to be told, "You have to wear it for two more weeks." So I wore this girdle for five weeks instead of two.

Waiting for the girdle to come off was an extremely difficult time for me. It was very painful, I think because of the trapped liposuction fluid and because the girdle was pressing on remaining breast tissue. This whole area continues to feel tight. I also have scars under my arms, not from the incisions, but from what I suspect was the spilling of liposuction fluid that was not wiped off properly onto my skin during surgery. These scars are like burns — I have lines and lines of burns on my back. When I showed them to the surgeon, he brushed off my questions by saying, "Put some vitamin E on it. It'll go away."

It's been almost three months now, though, and they have not gone away. Over time, the marks from the incision points have become darker. I also still have bruising on my chest, which I think is the result of the surgeon digging vigorously during the liposuction procedure to remove what he thought was fat. Of course, he didn't get "all the fat" because it wasn't all fat! He was supposed to remove actual breast tissue on my chest and he didn't.

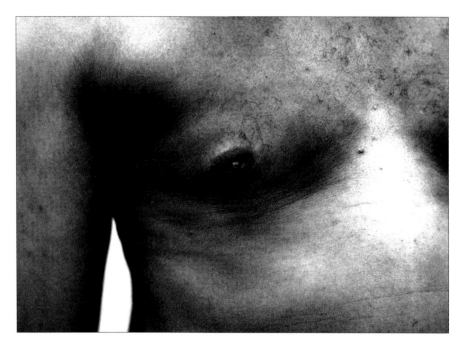

When I spoke to him about the bruising, he said, "It might go away, it might not, but that's life." When he said that, I thought, You know what? That's not good enough. I had waited a long time and was ready to sacrifice a place to eat, sleep and live to get rid of these things that were such an emotional burden to me. He acted as though what I was experiencing was trivial. I had paid good money for this surgery. If I had scars from breast removal incisions, I could accept them, because I'd been prepared for them. But I have no incision scars. I only have scars from liposuction entry points and from burns from liposuction fluid.

Since the surgery, I've gone back to see the surgeon five times. Each of these times, in addition to asking about the bruising and scarring, I have demanded that he remove the rest of the liposuction fluid. I've said to him, "Get the rest of this liposuction solution out." But he would only say, "No, no, wait until the girdle is off." Or later, "By now the body has dissolved

and absorbed it." In the end, he didn't take any action to resolve the fluid remaining in my chest. After I asked about the marks on my back many times, he finally said, "Come in at the end of October and we'll do laser treatments." I never did receive the laser treatments, though.

Pre-operatively the surgeon had informed me of the risks, but they hadn't included the things that happened to me. He never informed me about the possibility of skin discolouration, permanent bruising, or burns on my back. I continue to wonder if these reactions are the result of wearing the girdle too long.

My appointments with this surgeon never lasted more than five minutes. The last time I saw him, I took off my shirt for him to examine me. He reached for my waist, lowered my pants, and looked at my stomach. I asked, "What are you doing?" He said, "I think it looks very good." I said, "I did not have my stomach done."

He then looked at my chest and said, "You still have some scarring inside." I said, "That's not scarring, that's breast tissue! It's not a thick coating of skin or a thick under-skin. These are breasts." He had not removed the breast tissue; he'd simply removed the fat, leaving me with A-cup breasts. That's when I knew I could not trust this person to do anything more on me, including the laser treatments. He simply has an assembly line of people who want surgery to remove fat; people pay him, they are rushed through, and they have to deal with the consequences on their own. His specialty is breast surgery.

Since the surgery, I have also discovered that my breasts do not match — one is bigger than the other — and the nipples don't match either. One nipple protrudes and one is inverted. I'm pissed off about this. Both breasts, however, still come to a point, regardless of the nipples. I'm happy I don't have D-cup breasts, but I'm nevertheless back to square one. I cannot work out because my chest hurts too much. For example, if I jog, my breasts bounce, especially my left one, and the movement is painful. I'm not depressed, but I'm not pleased either, and I am going to do something about it. It was hard coming up with the money for the surgery and I didn't receive what I asked for. I don't see why I should live imprisoned by something that was not done properly.

I wear a single t-shirt now, because my breasts are not that big. I don't feel as self-conscious about them. I still have one big breast and one small one, though, and I can't raise my arms very high or extend my arms behind my back because of tightness in my chest. I think my skin might have bonded to my pectoral muscle. In fact if feels like my skin is ripping on the inside. So I know I need to see someone again.

I have decided I am going to seek new medical advice elsewhere, have the surgery redone, and bill the first surgeon for the second operation. The most important reason for the second procedure is to fully remove the breast tissue and to flatten my pointy breasts. I want the breast tissue out. I'm going to look for several medical opinions on how to proceed safely. I want to see someone who is reputable and experienced in doing corrective surgery.

I also decided to hire a lawyer, but before I did that, I needed to get more medical opinions. However, I didn't want to sue anybody. I didn't want to go through all that mess or have my experience be that public. In the end the lawyer told me my case would be a difficult one to win, and I would have had difficulty finding a new surgeon who would perform reconstructive surgery if a lawsuit were pending. In the end I chose not to proceed with a lawsuit. I haven't told anyone about the surgery until now. No one in my family, none of my friends — nobody knows I went through this.

I took a cab from the clinic instead of having someone pick me up. I looked after myself when I was laid up in bed for four or five days in a lot of pain. I took my dog out for walks on my own. Showering was the most painful thing because I couldn't raise my arms, but I didn't ask anybody to help me because I wanted this to be so private. My experience has been that, due to an unlikely combination of events, my body grew into what I felt was a deformity. And, if it's real to me, it's real.

I tried to correct a wrong — or correct something that made me uncomfortable — and I got butchered. I went in for surgery to correct one problem and I came away with several.

POST-SCRIPT
Two Months After the Second Surgery

I pursued consultation, and ultimately gynaecomastia surgery, with a second surgeon. The first surgeon, when I confronted him about having done liposuction instead of gynaecomastia, offered to re-do the surgery. I would have had to pay the hospital fees, but I didn't want to have this man cutting up my body. Originally he said he'd done "hundreds" of these procedures, but afterward he admitted that he'd done only "three on men." I found out from my second surgeon that liposuction can be a dangerous procedure. There is a risk of blood clots forming from broken blood vessels, which I wasn't told about the first time. And I didn't have a drain after the first surgery either, which should have happened. That's why the swelling was so severe. There was no way I was going to trust the first surgeon again.

After researching, I decided to drop the legal suit. I learned about others who had unsuccessfully tried to take this same surgeon to court. Because he's an MD, apparently he's entitled to perform the surgery, even though he isn't a specialist. Instead of going back to him, I paid $5,000 for the gynaecomastia. The second surgeon gave me much more information than the first one and a lot more support. It's been a really good experience.

The surgery has left my chest slightly asymmetrical and swollen. The swelling is supposed to go down within six months to a year. The incision was made around the nipple. I have no scarring at all, and the surgery was essentially painless. I took pain medications for a day or two and didn't need them after that. I had a drain for about five days, but it got blocked. On my first consultation after the surgery, the surgeon told me there was a blood clot in my chest and they had to go back in. That meant another general anaesthetic, and going under the knife one more time. Since then, some fatty tissue has developed on my pecs that I hope will go away. My second surgeon recommended I stay off steroids of any kind. Bruising on my back from the first surgery is still present and is likely permanent. The asymmetry might stay, but I won't know for sure until after a full year.

What can I say now? I've learned to live with what is left.

RECOMMENDATIONS

• Do as much research as possible about the procedure you're going to have. If you know what's supposed to happen, you're less likely to be taken in by someone who doesn't know, or doesn't have the experience.

• Do as much research as possible into your surgeon. Check his or her credentials. If you can, get a word-of-mouth referral. Some medical doctors who have not specialized in plastic surgery perform these surgeries and may not understand what you want. Ask if the doctor is affiliated with a professional plastic surgeon's association. Ask how many times he or she has performed this specific surgery.

EDITOR'S NOTE: All names have been changed to protect the identity of the participant and his family.

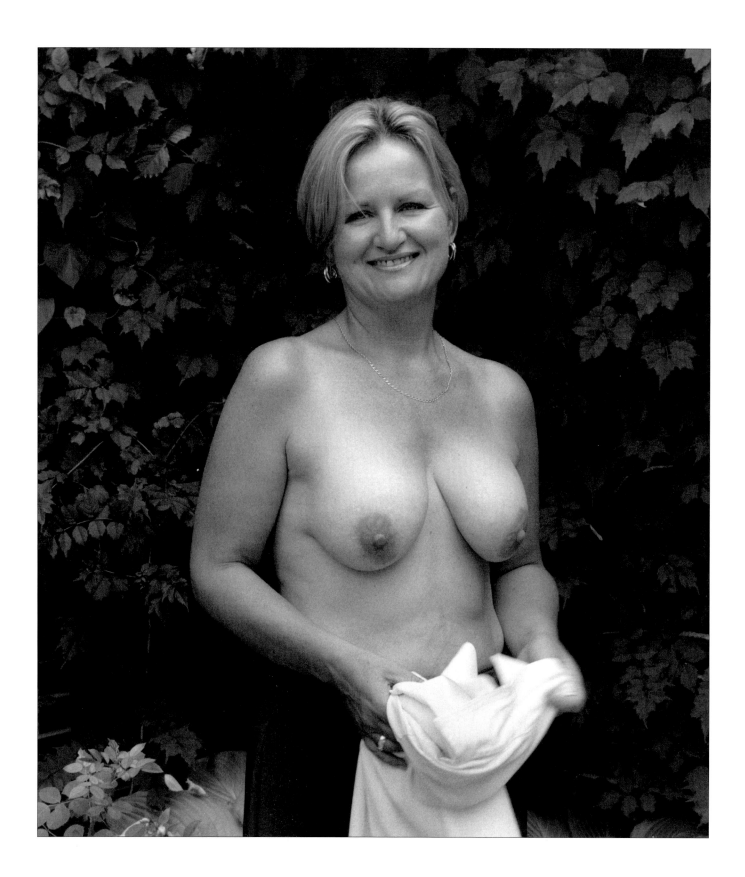

LAURA'S STORY
Discovering Myself

Laura had a breast augmentation with saline implants. The surgery was a choice she made as part of a process of self-discovery which included reclamation of her right to be a sexual being and enjoy her body. Laura's surgery took place in a whirlwind of change; she got the implants within months of her marriage ending, a tubal ligation surgery that went very badly, and the death of her mother. As a child, Laura lived in an environment of abuse. Although she has limited recall of the abuse, she believes this experience also had a significant impact on her surgical choice. She is thrilled with her implants. Laura is the mother of two children and sister to Angela, who is also part of My Breasts, My Choice. *Like Angela, she has maintained anonymity in her participation in the project.*

My breast augmentation surgery has been an integral part of a process of discovering my identity and allowing possibilities to come forth. I wrote this poem in January 1999, before the surgery and before some other important life-changing events had taken place.

> the back door flew open
> the wind blew in and rattled my bones
> I knew then that my heart needed to go
> to a warmer climate
> frozen over time
> icicles had imprisoned me
> but I'm thawing now
> the dark cave I enclosed myself in

> is slowly ravelling a path forth
> Sometimes when I try to emerge
> the sharp edges leave
> thin lines of pain
> across my back
> to get out
> I must allow some shards of ice in
> I know I can melt them, and
> emerge from this dark, cold
> empty place
> I believe

I'm not in that place anymore.

So many factors came into play when I was in the process of making the decision to have breast augmentation surgery. I had been talking about it with friends since I was in my thirties. I thought I would like having implants, but I didn't want to have the procedure because the silicone implants available at the time were known to be dangerous. Then, in the winter of 1998–99, a plastic surgeon spoke to a women's group I've belonged to for twenty years about saline implants. After his talk, I looked at the before and after surgery pictures he'd brought and thought, I want that! I felt brave. I was more in touch with my sexuality and felt better about my body image. I knew at this point that I was ready to have breast surgery.

This surgeon is the one I later consulted and had perform my augmentation.

In September 1998, my marriage ended and in February 1999, my by then ex-husband moved out. This spurred me on in considering augmentation. Then, on March 18, 1999, my mom passed away. Her death had the greatest impact on me, and altogether these experiences influenced my decision about augmentation. The whole process of making the decision became a spiritual journey for me. When I asked for guidance and clarity about which direction to go in, I received it. And I went with it. A new stage of my life unfolded from that point in the spring of 1999.

The time around the surgery was like a whirlwind. In addition to having a lot of clarity about things, I also felt a little manic. I was angry about so many things that had happened in my life. I probably weighed fifty pounds more than I do now. Every day, for years, I had been saying, I need to get out of here. I can't stand this any more. And then earlier in the fall of 1998 everything suddenly began falling into place. I started exercising, not to lose weight, but instead more as a shedding of my old self. I began to rediscover my sexuality, which had been shut down for my entire life, and to explore issues of body image. I was on a journey of self-discovery. It seemed as if things just began to unfold.

When my husband moved out, I felt as though I could finally begin to recapture myself. I'm not sure when I stopped being the old me, because I don't think I ever really knew who I was. I just knew I now wanted to find out. I was like a little girl in a candy store with all these choices. I had ended my marriage by saying, "You know what, I don't want to review this with you. I don't want to go anywhere. It's just over." I had such clarity in that experience.

I started to take baby steps forward. I got rid of a ton of shit including my marriage. It was a lot of hard work, but it was also amazing. I did a ritual cleansing. The ritual allowed me to get rid of a lot, including all the feelings I had about my marriage. Something really curious happened too. I had a cheap watch that had never worked and that the jeweller had refused to fix. In the midst of the cleansing ritual, it started ticking! Not everything felt comfortable, though, and for the longest time I couldn't sleep in my bedroom. I've only gone back to sleep in there in the last couple of months. Sometimes I really needed to be in the house alone, but with two kids, I didn't have the chance very often. When I was able to be alone, I sat on the floor and just rocked and rocked. I lit candles and let my grief come.

I feel fortunate that my mother was able to be supportive of me when I decided to walk away from my twenty-year relationship. Before she died, between September 1998 and March 1999, she became really gentle and extremely present as a mom for me. Never in my entire life had she been so unconditionally loving. There were no strings attached to her caring either — she just allowed things to happen. I would call her at ten o'clock at night or drive over, and I'd be weeping because, although it had been my decision to leave my marriage, I still needed to do all this grieving and let this go. My grieving and receiving her support were a big part of my starting to discover myself.

During this same period, the weight just came off and an attractive woman appeared. I didn't know who she was. People around me were shocked. They'd see me, and say, "Oh my god, you look good!" I liked that. I felt good. Men found me attractive. I felt like a fourteen-year-old. I felt like someone who had never had a chance to date, or explore sexuality, or have great sex. I had never let myself go to the place where you lose your mind in pleasure. I started to let myself go there and it was amazing.

In order to make the final decision about surgery,

I talked with different people. I talked with a friend who had implants, and I spent a lot of time talking with my sister Angela to help me make the decision. One day shortly after our mom died and before the surgery, Angela brought out a deck of women's tarot cards. I'd never done a tarot card reading before. We selected three cards: one for past, one for present and one for the future. My question was to our mom. I asked, "Do you think I should go ahead with the breast augmentation?" The first card I picked had on it a picture of a woman in a cave looking out, looking scared. That was my past card — it had the same images that I had in the poem I'd written. The second card, for the present, had a picture of a woman in front of a cave beside the tree of life. The third card, symbolizing the future, was beautiful. On it was a picture of a woman who was *full-breasted!* She was standing with her arms wide open, totally there. "Okay, now I know. You want me to do this. Thank you," I said to my mom. Angela and I just laughed. When I finally decided, *I think I'm going to do this,* both Angela and my friend were really supportive. The day I had the augmentation ended up being only weeks after my mom passed away. It felt sort of wild to have it happen that way. She passed away on March 18, and on April 24 I had my surgery.

Overall I received incredible support from the people in my life. I don't think I received anything negative, not once. No one ever challenged me about my decision to have augmentation surgery. Maybe that's part of my personality. When I make decisions in my life, I usually go ahead and implement them. And the people I surround myself with are a reflection of me: supportive and unconditionally loving. They did challenge me about certain things, but because I had been talking about augmentation for a long time, my friends knew how unhappy I'd been and how much it meant to me.

When I called the clinic to book the surgery, I put my name on the list for a cancellation spot — that's how much I wanted it done. I didn't doubt myself once. I just knew it was what I wanted, even though I made the decision to go through with it in such a short time span. I even paid for the surgery with my Visa card! I should have gotten travel points; then I could have gotten a trip out of it too!

Before the surgery, I went for an interview at the clinic. I picked up some information and told some more friends. My closest girlfriends, women that I have known for twenty years, helped me pick out my new size. I didn't want to go really big, but I did want to fill out the skin tissue. I had nursed both my children, and after losing weight I felt there was just nothing to my breasts any more. I also had a lot of stretch marks from the change in my weight.

The clinic let me take home different-sized implants. I was usually between a B and a B+, although sometimes I was a small C when I weighed more. I put the implants in my bra to see how much larger my breasts would feel. I like running and power walking, so I also ran with them in my bra. I bought some sweaters and blouses to try with them as well. How I would look was important to me. I didn't want to have people say, "That woman has implants. Look at those babies!" Now, with the implants, I'm a C. I discussed the size with the doctor. He did have some say in the decision because he refuses to put really large breasts on petite women like me.

Although it was important to get the surgeon's feedback, it was more important to get feedback from my friends. At one point I put some bigger implants in my bra, and I kind of liked them. I got a little excited and thought, Not bad! That's pretty big. Look at this sweater! But my friends said, "No, that's just too big." They talked me out of them, for which I am very grateful.

I had a tubal ligation quite unexpectedly before I

had my augmentation surgery. I had decided that I didn't want any more kids, and while I was waiting for an elective tubal ligation surgery date, one came up at the last minute. I ended up having two operations back to back.

Unfortunately, my tubal didn't go well. The surgical team lost a clip. Instead of ending up with a two-inch long incision, I ended up with one the length of a C-section. They had had to open me up further to look for the clip. The hospital staff said practically nothing to me about it. I was in recovery when the doctor who performed surgery came in. I asked her, "Is something wrong? I feel like I had a C-section." I was familiar with the feeling because one of my kids was born by C-section.

She said, "Oh no, I had to make the incision a little bit bigger." I finally saw it and it was ten inches long! Then no one called me back to have the staples that were used to close the incision taken out. When I went to the plastic surgeon's clinic for my breast surgery, I showed the nurse my stomach. By this time my skin had started to grow over the staples. The nurse said, "I was on the floor that day in the hospital. They shut everything down. They called everyone in and said, 'That'll never happen again.'" The surgical team had screwed up so badly that I guess the doctor didn't want to deal with me again and forgot to book an appointment for me to have my staples removed.

A nurse at the breast surgery clinic ended up taking out my staples. The breast surgeon couldn't believe I'd had them in for that long. I had no idea how long they should have been in or if in fact they were supposed to have dissolved. So I went into breast surgery while being in a state of shock. My sister Angela later said to me, "I thought the breast surgery wouldn't go well and the tubal would be fine." And it was the tubal surgery that ended up being messy. I did start to pursue a civil case about the tubal, but dropped it because I didn't have the energy for a legal battle.

As the day approached, I was very nervous about the surgery. On the morning of the operation I did some deep breathing to keep myself calm. It was still shocking the hell out of me that I was going to do this — just for me. I think that by having the surgery I was saying to myself, "You can do anything. You can take back your power. You can reclaim who you are. You can move forward in your life and do anything." At forty-one I was just beginning to feel these things.

I was impressed with the clinic where I had the augmentation. They were very professional. The surgical room in particular was better equipped than any hospital room I'd ever seen. It was sunny and cheerful. I had a sense that I was in good hands. I also received a top-of-the-line anaesthetic that was very clean and didn't leave me with the usual side-effects.

My surgery didn't take long. I went in at 7:30 a.m. was finished by 1:00 p.m. My girlfriend picked me up and took me home, where I rested. The next day, I went to stay with friends. For the next two weeks, I had a bit of bruising and swelling. Lifting my arms over my head was quite painful. I rested and took it easy. I'm not into taking lots of medication, so I took Tylenol 3 only on the first night and only took one round of antibiotics. The surgeon also told me he'd applied something internally to help fight infection, so I didn't anticipate any complications. The clinic staff outfitted me with a heavy-duty bra that I wore for the full recovery time of about six weeks.

The surgeon made very small incisions on the underside of my breasts where he inserted the implants. They're very little and almost gone now. At forty-one, I was too old to have the implants inserted under the muscle wall so instead I had them placed on top of the muscle wall. The surgeon created a pocket under my breast skin and fit the implant right up under my nipple. During this part of the procedure, the nerve endings sometimes get cut. I think this is how I lost sensitivity in my nipples. That's the only sad part for me about having had the surgery. I talked to several women who'd actually gained sensitivity. I have heard it's normal to lose some in the beginning after the surgery, but that it usually returns. I have gained only a small amount back. I don't like that. I have no sense of when my nipples are erect. During foreplay, I need more stimulation. I'd like to say, "Can you get a little rougher there? Here, use this sandpaper." I informed the people at the clinic of my condition and they were surprised, but it can be one of the consequences of getting implants. It can happen and it did happen to me. Women should think about whether they're willing to risk giving up sensitivity in their nipples if they are considering having breast augmentation.

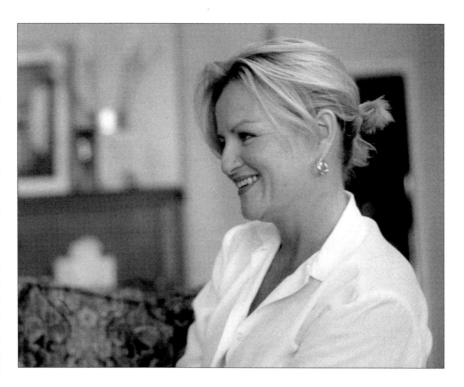

On the first night with my new breasts, I was afraid to look at them. The moon was full, however, and as I sat in my sunroom, I decided to peek. I took my sweatshirt off and lay flat, and there in front of me were these two mounds, these beautiful things. *Oh, my god! I have breasts!* I was so excited. It spurred me on to feeling a little more manic. I called the fellow I'd been dating, and he asked, "How are they?" "They're incredible. I lie on the floor and my breasts don't go anywhere!"

About a week later, he called and said, "Laura, come on over. I'm dying to see them."

I drove over. I felt a bit shy about them. I have always been shy about my body. I wore a big woolly sweater, as I was still not completely used to them, and I was still wearing the bandages. At that time, my breasts seemed huge to me, although they weren't.

I don't think I've dated anybody since who has ever caught on that I have implants. All they've ever said was, "Your breasts are beautiful." And I say, "Thank you." I never told any of them, except the fellow I was seeing at the time, about the surgery.

I progressed through the six-week recovery process of healing from both the tubal ligation and the breast surgery. My friends took me in and were really good to me. They put me in their guest room and babied me — brought me lunches, brought me magazines. I began to feel quite proud of my breasts. I was out on my friend's back deck one afternoon sipping a drink, and I asked my friend's husband, whom I've known for years, "What do you think?" He said, "Laura, it's not running season yet." I knew I had more healing to do before I could return to my regular exercise routine.

Right after my surgery, my breasts became engorged. The swelling went down after a month or two, but at the beginning they were quite swollen. I behaved a bit like a peacock, strutting around. I'd say to my girlfriends, "Look at this!" and then rip off my shirt to show them my breasts. I couldn't keep my mouth shut about them because I was so excited. I was also really open about the surgery. Of course, news can spread like wildfire and I hadn't realized how far it might go. I am sure there are some strangers who know me as "the woman with the implants." And I'm sure some people in the community made judgements about my choice. I'm much more discreet now. I don't walk around informing everybody I meet that I have implants and that it's the best thing that's ever happened to me.

Clothes have also been a big part of my self-discovery. Before the surgery, I used to wear baggy clothes that covered me up. I don't wear baggy things now but I wear don't clothes that are overly revealing either. I do like the fullness I have in my bra and under a sweater. My implants look really natural. When I have a bra on, my breasts look really sensual and really sexy, but I don't accentuate them by wearing low-cut things. It's just not my style.

Fortunately my implants don't make my breasts look like melons, as implants often do, because they lie right under the skin. Most often, implants are placed under the chest muscle wall, making the breast look larger and fuller. But because of my age, mine went in front of the muscle wall; my breasts hang from the weight of the implant. I wanted them to look natural. However, if I'm wearing a push-up bra, I notice the roundness of the implant shows. The implants haven't changed what physical activities I do at all, but when I'm doing them, my breasts do feel a little different. They ride up and down on my chest because of the way they have been inserted into a pocket of my skin.

Just recently I noticed that one breast is bigger than the other, so I'm going to be calling the surgeon to make sure everything is okay. It could mean anything. It could mean I have a slow leak. He needs to take a look. I'm not worried about it, because it's saline solution, and the body is supposed to absorb it. In terms of the health-related matters, I didn't worry too much. I realized that everything I read was going to be slanted depending on what study I was reading and who wrote it.

Initially I was very proud and really excited to have the implants. Now I don't even think about them, they're so congruent with my body. I would miss them terribly if for some medical reason I was told I shouldn't have them in. They've become a part of who I am — my breasts. My whole body is in sync with me, with the weight loss, the implants, exercising and self-care. If I get to choose, I'll have implants until the day I go. I'm not going without them!

I did decide to hide the surgery from my daughter, Megan. She still doesn't know that I had a breast augmentation. She was thirteen when I had it done. I know that period was a whirlwind for her, too — her mother and father split up; she lost her grandmother. For the first while, I wore sweatshirts around her because I didn't want her to catch on. I think she's still too young to notice because I think she sees breasts strictly as sex objects, and she might think of the surgery from that perspective. She might think, "My mom is sleazy" for making this choice.

I also wore an old swimsuit around her, one that didn't show much. Now I have a new swimsuit I like to wear, but around my kids I continued to wear the old one. I remember her looking at me once about two months after the surgery, a little confused, and she said, "Your breasts are big." And I said, "Yeah, they are." She said, "Oh." She still doesn't know. She's fifteen now. I'm going to wait till she's a young woman and then I'll tell her my story — when she's old enough to handle it. My son hasn't really noticed at all. He was ten at the time of the surgery, and it just didn't register with him. With my daughter it registered just a bit. She's starting to become full-breasted. Her close friends are beginning to say, "Megan, you're looking just like your momma."

The augmentation represented taking back many things, including making a decision solely based on me … People think of augmentation as something that will improve their sex life or their chances of getting a man. Part of my reason to have augmentation was so I would feel sexier, but mostly I was just so thrilled about making such an incredibly important decision for myself and going ahead with it. I felt brave and courageous.

I haven't always felt brave and courageous though. I have spent much of my life shut down.

Part of my shutting down and many of the life choices I have made have stemmed from the occurrence of incest in my family. I never really understood why I always felt different. I felt like I was on the outside of the circle looking in, never really part of life or that life flowed through me. I looked at people and thought, How can they just be silly and have fun? How can they just let loose? I was confused by how joyful people could be. I knew things were different for me, but I didn't understand why.

I don't actually have any memories of the incest in my family. All that I know is from the information that's been given to me. My older brother, John, told my sister Angela that he used to hold erections in front of me as a little girl and touch me sexually. He also disclosed that my father began sexually abusing me before I was a year old, when I was pre-verbal. My father would put a bureau in front of the bedroom door to keep anyone else out. One time my brother pushed it aside and saw me in the bed, my diaper off, with my father leaning over me as if he were performing oral sex on me. Often I woke up in other beds in the house and I never understood how I got there.

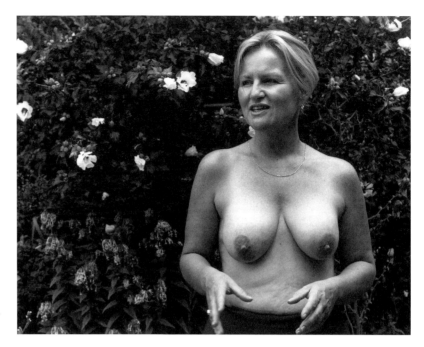

When the book *The Courage to Heal* by Laura Davis and Ellen Bass came out I was immediately drawn to it. I started to read and within a couple of pages, I had to vomit. I understood then that I had been a victim of childhood incest and that my body had known it for a long time, which was why I vomited. I have also known it consciously since I heard my brother John's disclosures. The place I emerged from as a child — a place of alcoholism, abuse and insanity in the household — I thought of as normal for a long time. I didn't know that that level of chaos and craziness wasn't normal.

Someone I was dating once said, "Someone told me that you're really messed up, that you are kind of slow and unable to follow things through." I could understand people thinking that. In my early twenties I had panic attacks but I had no idea where they stemmed from. I had difficulty concentrating or focusing and I couldn't study. I felt I couldn't get anywhere, so I underachieved for a long time. I had no idea what my potential was. I had no idea I was bright. I didn't even know that I could be articulate. Only now am I starting to think, Oh, my god. All of this is coming together for me. It's worked! I'm capable. I run this house. I make good investments.

I have worked hard to get from the place where I was in my early twenties to the place I am now. In my mid-twenties, I called a therapist and said, "I don't have an identity and I don't understand why." My healing took years before my life finally come together. Many things were taken away from me at such a young age. What went on in my childhood house was evil. I had no choice in the matter. I received no invitation that I could have accepted or rejected, but had to live through it.

My parents brought us up Catholic and used religion to teach us that sexuality was dirty. I remember keeping my sexuality hidden as a young person.

For years I had recurring nightmares related to the incest. They left me feeling horrible for days afterwards and I didn't understand where they came from. The nightmares started when I was maybe sixteen and continued into my late twenties. In them a dark, smelly presence would come down a hallway or up a set of stairs towards me, then I'd feel this breath — a deep breathing right beside me. The breath was very evil.

I have one very special memory and I believe it is of how I learned to cope with the incest. Our house backed onto a wooded lot, land that was supposed to have belonged to Native people. When I was maybe two or three, and for years afterwards, I remember I would wake up at night and go to the window. I would look out through the mist to the wooded lot and I would see about fifteen Native people dressed in feathers and beads standing together holding their drums. They would just be there. Then somehow they would come into the house and encircle my bed. They were my protection.

I developed another way to deal with my child-hood experiences and I remember it as the neatest thing. I used to leave my body at night. I had many of these out-of-body experiences as a young child, but I can't achieve them now as an adult. I've tried to, but I can't. I remember them as being so amazing! I would float down our huge slate front staircase, out the front door, and up above the house. Being up there in the darkness was beautiful for me. It was serene — I felt so free. In the first chapter of *The Courage to Heal,* the authors write about leaving your body as a way of dealing with the trauma of incest, and as a way of dealing especially with the trauma of the actual incestuous violation. That was the part in the book that made me vomit. Obviously I had understood as a child that something wasn't right. I had made a connection a long time ago, even though I don't have any exact memories of what it was. It's all written out for me in my body and in the book.

I believe that the incest, as well as my parents' alcoholism, especially my father's, and my father's physical assaults on my mother — all of it — set me up for the difficulties I have experienced as an adult. I'm now convinced that I have lost three of my four siblings because of our childhood suffering. In my late twenties, I had to walk away from my brothers, both of whom have unresolved psychological issues. Seeing their father sexually assault their infant sister — that has got to fuck you up. I lost my sister Christine, too. She committed suicide when she was twenty-seven. She talked about a rape and other incidents of abuse before killing herself. My family life was messy, really messy.

I think that, if there had been no incest, and if other structural things had been in place in our family that hadn't left us so isolated, things would have turned out much differently. If we hadn't had to keep family secrets and had been able to receive outside support or intervention, my sister might have survived and the rest of us might have fared better. My mom told me that during the sixties there were no women's shelters. Women didn't often leave abusive situations. In order to handle my father's beatings of my mother, I became a caretaker at a very young age. I ran around and wiped up the blood because I didn't want my other siblings to see it. My feeling was, I'd better clean up this mess. Well, I don't want any more messes in my life. I've chosen not to have any more messes. I refuse to have them. I'm tired of cleaning.

I get a little shaky when I talk about that particular part of my past. I don't go there very often any more. I feel like I've moved on. I want to honour that transition — my history *and* the moving on.

When I think about that time in 1999 I feel it was really too much — my mom's death, the end of my marriage, the tubal ligation, the augmentation — all of it. I don't feel the same way now as I felt at the time of my breast surgery because things have calmed down. I've slowed down. My plate's not so full, and I am focussing on my children. At the time of the surgery I was "out there" somewhere. Now I'm back with both feet planted firmly on the ground. I know where I'm going, and I'm there 150 percent for my kids.

I've arrived. Not quite full circle, because I've never been here before. Rather I have arrived at a new place, and I like who I am here. I am grateful for the gifts I have received. For me my implants, and the strength I had to make the decision to get them, were a gift.

Recommendations

For me the decision to have augmentation surgery was a very personal one. I want other women to know the decision has to come from within them, and not from a mate saying that he'd like her to have bigger breasts. A woman needs to feel that augmentation will complement her total being. It has to be a fit for the whole person. If augmentation is something that she has thought about for a long time, if it's been a dream, it can be worth pursuing.

Once she has decided to have an augmentation, I think it's important she choose a breast size that is congruent with her body type. It is also important to research your surgeons, and get good recommendations from other people. I suggest going to Web sites, talking with other patients, and getting feedback. I did that. For example, I read stories about women who chose implants that were too large and ultimately had to go back for surgery to reduce them.

I gathered quite a lot of information before the surgery. I read through it carefully and made sure I was fully aware of the risks. Implants usually last eight to ten years before they need to be replaced. Sometimes they need to be replaced before then because they break.

The replacement surgery is less expensive though because the pockets are already there. The surgery is not as intrusive, but it is still full surgery involving a general anaesthetic.

If I wanted to, I could choose breast-lift surgery next time, to make my breasts look perky, but I'm not sure it's important for me to do that. Bras can do that. This way, I will sag just like any other woman. From what I've heard, the lift is not actually very pleasant and it creates quite a bit of scarring.

I recommend massaging the implants on a daily basis to keep them from hardening. The clinic staff also recommended always wearing a bra to support the weight of the implants. I wear my bra all the time, including to bed. I haven't had a mammogram since the implants, so when I book my physical I'll inform them. The radiologist will need to know I have implants to read the results accurately.

EDITOR'S NOTE: All names have been changed to protect the identity of the participant and her family.

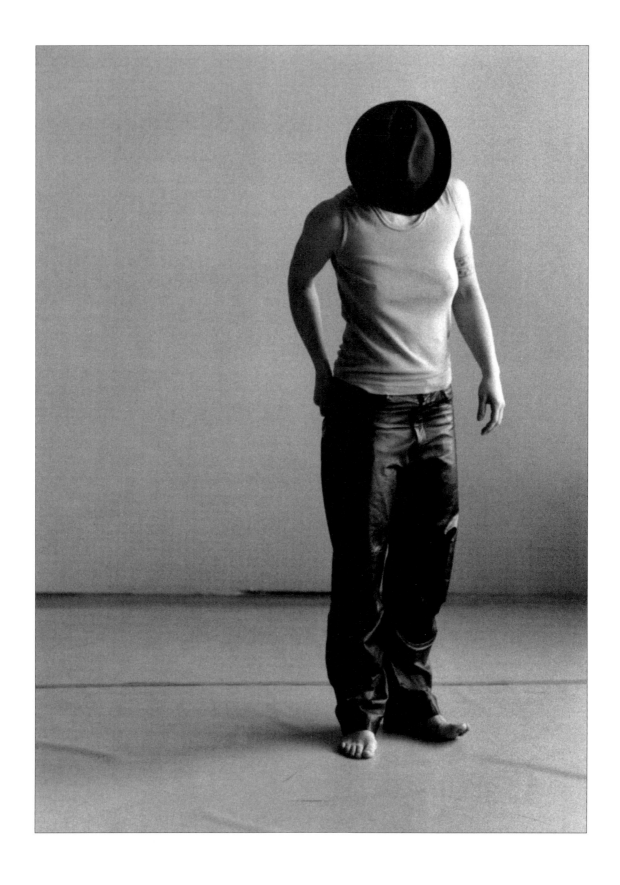

CORRIN ADAMS
Reclamation and Acceptance

At sixteen, Corrin Adams, experiencing the limitations of societal gender expectations, sought freedom of movement and self-expression in part through breast reduction surgery. At the time, the surgery was an empowering choice for Corrin. Since the surgery, the scars have continued to become inflamed. Over the last ten years Corrin has moved through doubts and regret about her surgical decision to come to a place of self-acceptance. She is currently in the process of tattooing her breasts as another measure of reclaiming her body as an expression of her self. She enjoys challenging culturally defined male and female physical images, playing with gender representation while experiencing and naming herself totally as woman.

Corrin is a dancer, yoga instructor and fine-cuisine caterer. She is interviewed by My Breasts, My Choice *editor Barbara Brown.*

CORRIN: I had a breast reduction ten years ago. I had to wait until my seventeenth birthday. I made my decision to have a breast reduction when I was sixteen, and I made it really quickly. Since the surgery, I have had a hard time coming to grips with the decision. For a long time I thought I was really vain: *I'm a bad woman.* I'm a bad feminist. I'm a bad lesbian. I questioned how I could have made this choice to alter my body cosmetically. How could I have given control over my body up to a man, to a male surgeon who's going to use my body, who's going to make decisions about what he thinks looks good? And, he's going to make tons of money off me.

BARBARA: How did you begin thinking about having breast reduction surgery?

CORRIN: I have no idea. Obviously I was young and I think I was still developing physically. I don't know how it came into my head — probably through magazines. Somewhere I found out the surgery was covered by OHIP [Ontario Health Insurance Plan] and so it made the choice possible. I didn't have it because I wanted to fit in with what the social idea of beauty is. I realized having the surgery was a way for me to control my body. It's almost like I don't relate to the person that I was when I made that decision.

Even right after the surgery it was really hard for me to know what I was thinking, because it didn't change my body that much. I think he took less than a cup size away. The surgeon decided that if he took any more away I would look out of proportion and I wouldn't have the right aesthetic for a woman. I was disappointed after the surgery, realizing that I still had breasts. I realize now that in reality I just didn't want them at all. I wanted him to make me a flat-chested woman. I wanted to be able to do sports, and I wanted to be able to speak my mind and not feel like my breasts were interfering. I wanted to be androgynous, but that didn't happen.

BARBARA: How was it that the surgeon made the choice about size?

CORRIN: He made the decision during surgery. There wasn't a lot of talk beforehand about what I could expect. I didn't even know what the scars were going to look like. I never saw any pictures — of his work or pictures of any woman who'd had the surgery. I'd never talked to anybody who'd had it. I saw the surgeon twice. In the first meeting, which was very short, he set up a file and he briefly described the procedure. I remember leaving feeling unclear about what would happen. Visual aids such as photographs were something I would have wanted in order to feel more clear. In the second meeting, I took my shirt off and he drew with marker all over my bare chest in preparation for the surgery. Given all the lines drawn on my chest, I didn't know where the cuts would be made.

BARBARA: How did you find your surgeon?

CORRIN: I went to a walk-in clinic and said that I was having back problems and that I wanted to have a breast reduction. The doctor then referred me to a surgeon.

BARBARA: Did you have photographs taken?

CORRIN: When I got my blood tests at the hospital, a nurse took two photos. I remember nobody talked to me. I was sort of shuffled in and out.

BARBARA: Do you remember how you felt during that process?

CORRIN: I think because I was so young and hadn't yet taken full control of my own health and overall well-being, that I didn't know what to expect from modern medicine or doctors. I didn't expect to have anything more than I was given, so I just went along with everything that happened.

BARBARA: Did anyone influence your decision?

CORRIN: I was living with my mom at the time and she didn't say much about it. I did talk to one friend of hers who's a referee and into sports. She said she would have had the surgery when she was younger if she'd had that option. She felt that her breasts got in the way and hindered her position as a referee and a sports teacher. She also felt that, because of her breasts, she didn't get the respect she deserved generally. I don't know if this is true, but part of me feels that maybe my mom thought it was a bit of a novel idea. What I got from her — and this was the same no matter what I did — was basically, "It's your life, it's your body, and that's all I have to say."

BARBARA: Was your mother's permission necessary to have the surgery at that time?

CORRIN: No, but I still had to wait for my seventeenth birthday. That was the only condition given to me by my referring doctor, in adherence to medical guidelines. I was very young to have been having surgery that was so extreme. I know a lot of people do extreme things to their bodies whether they are young or not, but I think it's ridiculous that society is so accepting of it as a form of self-mutilation without acknowledging it as such.

BARBARA: What was the recovery process like for you?

CORRIN: My recovery was very quick. I'm sort of a fighter. It was as quick as making the decision and going through it. I was pretty sick afterwards from the anaesthetic though: I remember vomiting a lot right after the surgery. I was in a lot of pain overall. The nurses were trying to give me painkillers, but I didn't want them. Going through the recovery process without painkillers was something I needed to do. The nurses didn't come the second day. I think they were pissed off that I wouldn't take the pills.

On the second day after the surgery, the surgeon came in and took the dressings off and showed some other guy in a white jacket. They both looked at my breasts and said, "Yes, it's a good job." The surgeon had pulled the bandages up so I couldn't see. He redressed it, and I never saw the surgeon again.

I remember being excited at this point in the recovery. *I'm not going to have any breasts in a week! It's just the swelling.* When I finally took the bandages off, however, I still had them.

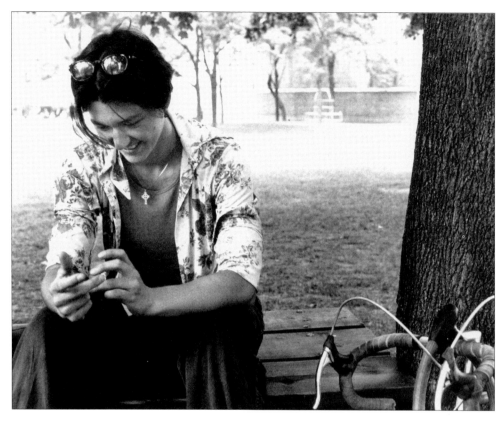

The whole thing was a very, very solo undertaking. I realize that I took myself, emotionally and physically, to a very isolated place before and after the surgery. I didn't tell my dad; a lot of other people didn't even know. I was out of school for a week and when I went back, I told everybody that I'd been sick. They told me I looked ten pounds thinner. That satisfied me and I just jumped back into my life.

BARBARA: Did the reduction change your activities or lifestyle?

CORRIN: I felt a little more confident about what I wore. I didn't have to think about it so much. I hadn't liked attention paid towards my breasts, so after the surgery, I felt a little more in control of that attention. I felt like my breasts were less of a draw. I would have liked them to be even less so, but it *was* better.

Dealing with the scars was another issue altogether. I wouldn't change in front of anybody. Taking my shirt off in front of others — peers and lovers — was difficult because it made me confront my decision and forced me to take responsibility in a way I wasn't ready to. I was very self-conscious about them. I wouldn't change in front of anybody. I went through many head-trips about the scars.

I went to Michigan Womyn's Music Festival for the first time not long after I had the surgery. I was eighteen. Walking around with all those women who to me seemed so natural and beautiful made taking my shirt off there a huge step.

BARBARA: And what were you in comparison to them?

CORRIN: I was wounded. I was damaged goods. Not so crass as "goods," but I had been through stuff and I felt it was obvious. Sometimes I rationalized the choice and the experience by fantasizing that some guy had attacked me with a knife, and the scars were what he had left behind. I held on to that fantasy for a while and it made me feel better.

BARBARA: What did the fantasy give you?

CORRIN: I could let go of the responsibility for having altered my body. That was the hardest thing, acknowledging that I had made that choice.

BARBARA: What did it mean for you to have made that choice, the choice to have breast surgery?

CORRIN: Well, I thought of myself as being marked by my choice; it was like I had this huge sign across my chest. When I looked in the mirror, it read, "You're not capable of accepting yourself" and "You're vain." I felt like I had betrayed the whole female race.

BARBARA: By making this choice?

CORRIN: Yeah. I felt I had betrayed myself, and betrayed every other woman who deals with any kind of physical challenge. I had a perfect body. There was absolutely nothing wrong with it, and I went and had cosmetic surgery to alter it.

BARBARA: Does that feeling of self-betrayal remain for you now?

CORRIN: No, no.

BARBARA: How did it change?

CORRIN: For the longest time I held on to that feeling. I always said to women who complained about their breasts, "Accept yourself. You're beautiful. Learn to love your body. Find ways to cope and find ways of being in your body where you can support the weight of your breasts no matter what you're doing."

But now, hearing other strong, amazing women talk about their thoughts about breast reduction and not hide it has been really great. Just the fact that I've been able to talk about my breast reduction for this project has been really great. Talking with other women has also helped me realize what I was seeking — androgyny — and that I wanted people to see me as *me* first not female first. Realizing that what I'd wanted were *no* breasts is a pretty recent realization. Having talked to other women who share that desire, I wonder if removing one's breasts will become something that women opt for in the future by means of elective surgery.

BARBARA: Does that desire for androgyny mean you have questions about gender identity?

CORRIN: No, I don't. I don't feel any less a woman, nor any desire to identify as anything other than a woman. I think that my breasts defined me as I grew up. It separated me from the boys and made me have to deal with hassle.

BARBARA: So your choice towards having no breasts, being flat-chested, is a choice related to wanting less hassle — freedom?

CORRIN: Yeah, physical freedom — the freedom to be able to put on shorts and a t-shirt and walk out the door and not worry that people might stare at my breasts — the freedom to be able to use my chest as a breastplate rather than as something to be hunched over. Women are often protecting themselves when they hunch over their chests whereas men can use their chests like a breastplate to approach life confidently. I admire women who have that kind of confidence and openness in their chests and in themselves and are able to maintain it.

I think, more than anything else, more than feeling free by the size of my breasts, I just feel free by having focused on them for so long and so intensely.

BARBARA: What kind of freedom have you gotten from focusing on them?

CORRIN: I don't feel they're private anymore. I remember walking into a dance class one time in a teeny little see-through Snoopy tank top. My breasts were falling out every time I bent over. I didn't think about it at all, even though I didn't know any of those people. The other day I went running and did 10 K. I realized when I got to the ravine that I had forgotten to put a bra on. That is what I've always wanted: not to have to worry. And when I'm boxing or dancing, I rarely wear a bra either.

Certainly I go through phases where I am more self-conscious about my breasts than at other times, but for the most part I'm not self-conscious at all. I think I am becoming less and less afraid of losing parts of myself. I am more accepting of my choices. I'll never be a guy. I hate to say it, given we're in very modern times, but it's like penis envy — pectoral envy — and envy of the cockiness that comes with it, the right to take up space. I don't know yet how I will make my way to feeling fully confident in my body.

Before I had the surgery, I was having a hard time asserting myself and I felt like my sexuality was at the forefront of everything I did. I wanted to get rid of the barrier it created. I felt out of control. But after the surgery when I went back to school, I was able to use my sexuality. I went back totally decked out, feeling thinner and less busty, and wearing tight shirts. I was able to be more flamboyant, which is what I wanted to be. I wanted to be able to be anything and not feel trapped by my body. I wanted freedom, and I felt that with a super-feminine body I didn't have that freedom. I felt I couldn't play one role and then another and expect to receive full respect and acceptance for being either one.

BARBARA: What's your reflection on the factors that influenced you feeling out of control?

CORRIN: I think that those factors have to do with my upbringing, being brought up by a single mom whom I didn't see as having a strong sense of power about her. I felt she set limits on herself that I didn't want set on me. I felt restrictions placed on me socially and culturally that made me feel frustrated and angry. I felt, Okay, some actions are going to have to be taken here because I'm not satisfied with the roles available to me. At that point, I saw myself with two options. I could be submissive, motherly, feminine and frumpy — a sort of housewife or martyr. Or I could be the all-powerful James Bond diva and use my sexuality to its utmost.

But I didn't think I could be this James Bond diva if I had really big breasts because they would get in the way. If I were running naked across the desert with a gun, I couldn't have my breasts flailing all over the place. I've been training as a dancer since I was two. I was born with a strong physical structure and as a dancer, I work with that. Gender roles were and are frustrating. I wasn't interested in being a passive female. My big-screen image of what being passive meant was of someone who is quite aimless. I wanted to be an Olympic gold-medal achiever. I wanted to be something — a superpower hero. Something good. Something strong.

BARBARA: So the surgery made the possibilities of how you expressed yourself across expected gender roles wider?

CORRIN: Definitely. I think a part of me also felt empowered by actually having made the decision and gone through with it. It astounds me how little fear I had about the surgery.

BARBARA: Was there any point at which you felt a lot of fear?

CORRIN: Remorse. I never felt fear. With these scars, I believed I could never have my innocence again. I had taken away my own innocence. I felt guilty for doing that to myself and for putting myself through something that I didn't necessarily have to go through. Because, for me, having breast surgery wasn't about improving my health, it was about changing my body. I put breast reduction on a par with things like tattooing or modifying a body in other ways. I think this connection is a very contemporary idea. I know that people have been altering their bodies in different ways for centuries, but this choice, cosmetic surgery, is a contemporary one.

My desire for the longest time — for years, for years — was wishing that I had not made that decision at all, wishing I could have my breasts back. Why? Because I didn't want to have the scars. I didn't want the responsibility. It was a desire for a return to my natural, untouched state. I felt like I had betrayed the whole woman race. Back then I felt regret at not being able to move forward; not being able to talk to myself and ask, Why? I would really like to work with myself as I was then. I'd say to myself, So many people have way larger breasts than you do. Your best friend has way larger breasts than you do. What makes it so important for you to have this done, that you need to have this kind of control? Why are you taking this direction as opposed to other things that give you control in your life? I'd give myself the support that I didn't have then.

I was pregnant a while back. My breasts got bigger. I loved it. They were reminiscent of the size they had been. I finally felt what that would be like, having my breasts back, and I really enjoyed it.

BARBARA: Do you ever ask yourself if you should have made a different decision?

CORRIN: Oh, yeah. For a long time I regretted making the decision to have breast reduction. I ask myself that a lot of times, and I always say that I would not have had the reduction had I known anything, had I talked to people about it. I had inadequate information to make an informed choice.

BARBARA: What would you have wanted to know before you made your choice to have reduction surgery?

CORRIN: What I really wanted, even then, was to see pictures of the scars. I wanted to know what they would look like. In the appointment before the surgery, the surgeon said, "It'll be like this, and like this, and like this," making marks on my body. That was two days before the surgery and I was meant to keep the marker on my body. This was going to be his tool, his diagram for where to cut.

As he was putting this permanent marker on my chest I couldn't even look. I felt like a vulnerable little girl. There was marker everywhere, so I had no clue where the cuts or scars were going to be. I didn't know how deep they would be. I didn't know what it would look like five years down the line. I also wasn't given any information about how to take care of the incisions or the scars. I would have liked to have had more information about these things.

BARBARA: What did you do after the surgery in terms of self-care for a return to health?

CORRIN: I think I just did the basics. They probably gave me a course of antibiotics, and if they did, I took them. I lost sensation in the nipples. During the surgery the whole nipple is taken off, so the nerve endings are cut, and then the nipple is placed back on — cut and paste. For a while after the surgery I basically had no sensation in my nipples. The incisions

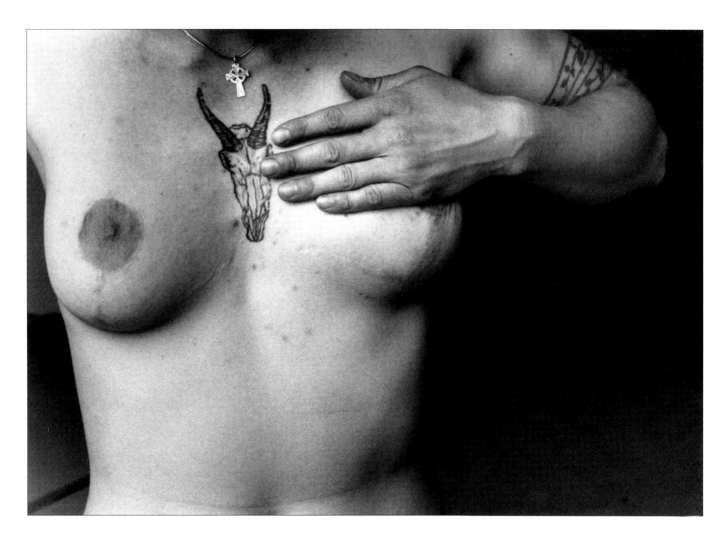

healed, but they still get inflamed a sometimes.

BARBARA: Has any of the sensation in your nipple come back?

CORRIN: The sensation has definitely developed and come back a lot although it's difficult to remember the extent of sensation I had before the surgery. My nipples won't stay erect for very long. During sex that makes me feel inadequate in a way; I don't look turned on. I have to fake it. I think it's so beautiful — women who have super-hard nipples — it's gorgeous. I've always wished I had that. I have so many "I wish, I wish."

BARBARA: Do particular things bring on the inflammation on?

CORRIN: No, not really. Some points along the incisions didn't close fully when the stitches dissolved and these areas are still very susceptible. They fill up with pus sometimes, and that's gross, but nothing in particular seems to bring this reaction on.

BARBARA: How do you deal with it?

CORRIN: I take a bath and moisturize my body and try to treat it with extra care. Sometimes I'll massage oil into my nipples and scars. The massaging is more for emotional nurturing than anything else.

BARBARA: Have you noticed any other physical changes since the surgery?

CORRIN: I've noticed and thought about a couple of things. I don't know if this can be proven, but my body seems to have formed around having smaller breasts. I was a bigger person before. The breast reduction seems to have reduced my whole body size.

I also think the surgery affected my immune system. What got me thinking about this was when a dog bit me once and I ended up with red streaks going up my arm and into my breast. My breast was huge and swollen, and I ended up in the hospital for a month. I had blood poisoning, but I wonder if having had the breast tissue taken away affected how long it took for me to get over the bite. It makes me wonder.

BARBARA: What support would you want someone in a similar position to receive?

CORRIN: I think that I would have really liked acceptance, support that wasn't biased. For a long time, I was biased and would have said to others, "Don't. It's wrong. It's purely cosmetic. It's pure vanity." I would have liked to have talked to someone who was willing to discuss the choice and to give me as much information as possible. That's what I was lacking: information. But at that age, who among us has a community that could support or talk about a decision like that? What sixteen-year-old can go to her friends and say, "I've decided to have a breast reduction. What do you think? Can we talk about this?"

I think that people should be counselled on the scars before they go through with it. I think that if what they're after is a greater self-acceptance by having breast surgery, they've got to be aware that every time they look in the mirror, they're going to have this huge, gashing reminder. With breast reduction, the scars are not small. They pretty much cover most of your breast surface and they're not ever going to go away. I think it is quite important for people to be aware of the scarring they'll have.

BARBARA: Do you think that responsibility to counsel lies within the women's community, within the medical establishment? Where would you have wanted that to happen?

CORRIN: For sure, I think it lies in both. For a long time I was, and am still, definitely very angry about the fact that, I'd say, 99 percent of cosmetic surgeons are men and, I'd say, probably 99 percent of the people who get cosmetic surgery are women. I think that is a pretty important statistic to think about.

BARBARA: How did that gender dynamic affect you at seventeen, when you went for your surgery?

CORRIN: I didn't expect much. Now I have no idea who the surgeon was, what his name was. I don't have any records or source for his accountability. I remember wishing that he would give me a list of women I could call who were willing to talk about their experiences. But I don't think many male surgeons would ever do that. He certainly didn't. I remember wanting to talk to the doctor's secretary, but she didn't have anything to say. She didn't communicate with me beyond what was necessary to set up a file.

I would have liked to have seen a book of photos of his work, like when you go into a tattoo shop. I would have liked to have been able to say, "This is what I want to get out of this. I have a C cup, and I'm not going through a $5,000 surgery and putting my body through huge trauma and all this medicine to get a B cup. I also think I should have been sent to a shrink to at least talk it out. I wouldn't have wanted the shrink to get rid of my desire or to convince me to change my decision, but I would have liked to talk it out. I think that if I had been able to talk it out, I could at least have made a more informed decision.

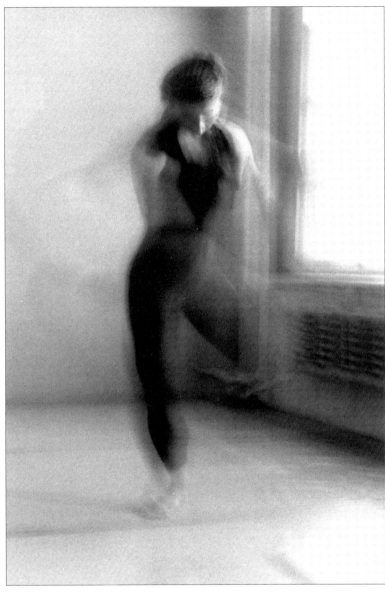

helped me gauge my comfort level with those people, so that was good in a way. I was very cautious for a long time, but now I'm very, very open. It was interesting to realize that people generally didn't notice. I'm also usually in environments that are supportive. Interestingly, five years ago the scars were less visible than they are now because I've lost weight and my pecs are stronger. This means my breasts sit higher and the scars are more visible.

My scars, my choice, have become a part of who I am. One summer at the Michigan Womyn's Music Festival a few years ago, a woman brought out a remedy to diminish and heal scars even if they were really old. I looked at it and thought, "Oh, that's very cool," and it didn't even occur to me at the time that I had any scars on my body to apply it to. They've become very much a part of my body.

I've very recently come to a point where I feel like I'm going to use tattooing to incorporate the scars into something beautiful.

BARBARA: How do you think getting tattoos will play itself out in your life? What will it mean?

BARBARA: Even if it was the same decision?

CORRIN: Yeah.

BARBARA: How do you feel about your scars now? What's your comfort level in being naked by yourself, with a lover, or changing at the pool?

CORRIN: With lovers it took a long time to feel comfortable. How I felt about sharing my scars with them

CORRIN: I think getting them is about reclaiming my beauty. It's going to take a while to decide on the tattoo design because I am becoming more specific now about what I think is beautiful, what qualities I love and want to develop in myself. My body is a palette. "This is my body. This *is* my body." That's profound for me. It's the difference between this being my body in its unnatural form — which is how I thought of it, me being separate from my body — and realizing that my body is an expression of who I am and where I've been.

I can now take responsibility for having had the surgery; it means I can accept myself, love myself, nurture myself. If I ever feel uncomfortable, that's okay — I know I can go through that with myself. In order to do all this, though, I've really had to slow down, slow way down in my relationship with myself.

BARBARA: Do you think that your choice to have breast reduction was a step into your body, into yourself?

CORRIN: Sort of, in a roundabout way. Definitely I made it in an effort to connect with myself, but in a very controlling way, not in a supportive way. I can see now that for example the way I dealt with myself after the surgery was very harsh, very brash.

BARBARA: You called the surgery "mutilation." Is that what it feels like for you?

CORRIN: Yes. I don't judge myself for it, but I don't have any coddling affirmations for myself about it either. I accept that at that point in my life, the decision was an important one. Over time I'm realizing all the different implications it has had. It wasn't only about altering my feminine aesthetic; the decision was also connected to my sexuality. It was about a whole lot of other things. Talking to women recently about breast reduction surgery has helped me to remember all the reasons I was adamant about the decision. I was adamant to the point that I put myself through a very extreme type of surgery without any information or any support, or even anyone questioning me either. The decision wasn't made in a fury.

I went through a lot of head trips because I felt isolated and I didn't have the amount of support I would have liked from others. I don't feel I was very self-supportive, and at seventeen, I wasn't able to ask for what I needed. So I guess that brings me back to what I would want for others who are thinking about surgery. I'd want them to nurture and be soft with themselves, physically and emotionally. Providing support has nothing to do with influencing people to make specific choices; I think it just helps people develop a capacity for self-acceptance, to accept that, no matter what, this is the only body we've got.

So, I think, to get my breasts — my scars — tattooed is a kind of reclamation, a way of saying, You're so awesome that not only do I accept your scars, I'm going to make them beautiful. I'm going to give this to you and we're not going to feel shame about it. We're not going to hide the fact that you have scars. We're going to embellish them and really embrace that area of your body instead of constantly hiding it — which is what I did before and after the surgery. It's a way to give myself a gift. I think that the best possible outcome is where I am right now.

PART II

THE JOURNEY TO HEALING
Health Care

Peer Support: Empowerment for Choice

Pauline Bradbrook

A diagnosis of breast cancer is an overwhelmingly frightening experience. A cascade of emotions runs riot: fear, disbelief, anger, grief, loneliness. At the same time, decisions need to be made. One of the first decisions we face with this diagnosis is a surgical one. Will the surgery be removal of the tumour and surrounding tissue (a "lumpectomy" or partial mastectomy), possibly followed by chemotherapy, radiation and hormonal therapy? Or will the surgery be removal of the breast itself (mastectomy), possibly followed by the previously mentioned treatments? Will there be axillary lymph node dissection? Will there be breast reconstruction of some type, and if so, will that be immediately after surgery or will it be delayed? These choices bring us face to face with our own mortality.

Sometimes there isn't actually much of a choice. In my own case, the cancer was too extensive to be treated by a lumpectomy. My surgeon strongly recommended a modified radical mastectomy with axillary node dissection. There was really no choice, though immediate breast reconstruction was offered as an option. I made a choice against reconstruction.

I grew up with horror stories about women who went into surgery for removal of a breast lump, only to wake up and find that their breast had been amputated. There was no choice related to the surgery, nor any real consent to the procedure. Those days are not all that distant. I remember, for example, that two of my aunts had radical mastectomies. Even just a few decades ago, in most of the country there was no option for breast reconstruction either. A breast cancer diagnosis left a woman in a situation where there was nowhere to turn for information or support from others who had experienced this health crisis. Power was strictly in the hands of the medical professionals, who held the information. The deep loneliness and shock that is inherent in such a diagnosis and the accompanying surgery were exacerbated by the lack of emotional connection with others who had had the same experience.

Organizing and political action have done much to alter this scenario for many breast cancer patients. Currently, many women (or men) are given a choice between having a lumpectomy followed by standard treatments, or having a mastectomy, which may also be followed by additional treatment. Presently, in cases of mastectomy, a patient often has a choice for breast reconstruction either concurrently with the mastectomy or later. Increasingly, peer support counselling and peer support groups are available to provide support in the decision-making process.

Peer support is fundamentally about empowerment through sharing of experience and information. It can be offered informally without an organizational context, via the Internet, for example; or formally, through services offered by non-profit organizations such as Willow Breast Cancer Support and Resource Services, Wellspring, or the Canadian Cancer Society, who have guidelines and principles governing the services.

At Willow, for example, telephone support is available on a toll-free basis for callers from across the country, in addition to drop-in support for individuals living in or visiting Toronto. Peer support volunteers and staff, all of them survivors, are trained intensively in the latest information on breast cancer and its treatment. Packages of information tailored specifically to each individual's needs are offered to those who wish them. While Willow does not run breast cancer support groups, it does provide support for those who wish to get a group going in their community. They also refer callers to the Canadian Cancer Society and other agencies which do offer support groups. Breast cancer support groups have multiplied in recent years across the country, and many people find meeting regularly with peers profoundly helpful for emotional support and shared information.

Who is a peer in your situation? An easy answer might be anyone who has needed a modified radical mastectomy. Is it important for a peer to match you in age, gender, race and sexual orientation as well? My own experience as a breast cancer survivor and peer support counsellor is that these vital factors in our situations do influence the way in which peer support is experienced. I respond to calls from women who are eager to speak with someone who has experienced exactly their own diagnosis and treatment recommendation, but socio/cultural connections are also prominent. I could provide important information to a young gay male breast cancer patient, for example, but I would not likely be perceived as a peer in terms of the experience. It helps enormously to know how a peer made her decisions, how treatment was experienced, and what quality of life has resulted. Hope springs from talking to a peer who has survived. It is also important to be clear about how individual the experience of breast cancer treatment is. My experience may not be yours, which is why it is most beneficial to connect with more than one experience.

Ideally, peer support is a non-directive and non-judgmental activity. It is based in the belief that a fully informed person ultimately knows what is best for her or him. As a peer support counsellor, my role is to provide accurate information and to support the caller in the choices she makes. A non-directive approach requires that I never advise a caller what to do, even when this is precisely what she wants. My role is to create opportunities for the caller to gain new insights into her situation and enable her to make a decision that fits for her. My hope is that, as a result of our conversations, she feels less isolated, and is empowered to make her treatment choices.

PAULINE BRADBROOK has been active in feminist issues for many years. Her career focus has been theological education for ministry. Currently, she is employed as a peer support counsellor at Willow Breast Cancer Support and Resource Services, Toronto.

The Transition:
Transsexual and Transgendered Peer Support

Christina Strang

Being transsexual is one of the most beautiful things in the world. We are not freaks; we are a beautiful unique people with a culture and history that expands and covers every religion, ability, class and country on this planet. There are realities in our communities that need to be addressed about poverty, HIV/AIDS prevalence, sex-trade workers' rights, transitioning support, surgical choices, isolation, and lack of accessible trans-informed literature and health care. It is said that in transsexual and transgender people, self-esteem is the number one motivation behind high-risk behaviour. I have to say that we are all incredible, beautiful creatures — and with our self-esteem in high gear, the high risk is with the barriers that oppose us. Fight for your health, fight for your community, and fight for the cause.

Peer Support Program Development

Peer support, formally and informally, is a primary tool for shifting these realities. Community-based efforts are part of a growing trend in social services to serve marginalized populations through peer support programs. The peer support philosophy is to hire and promote skill development to empower a community to better serve themselves and advocate for their own needs. Peer support programs do not necessarily hire trained therapists or counsellors, but rather hire trained therapists or counsellors, but rather individuals who come with experiences similar to those faced by participants. Those involved work actively in their communities to share information, provide a friendly ear and shoulder, and bring a commitment to empower others like themselves with a sense of pride and healthy self-esteem.

In the program I work with, we hire transsexuals who have valid sex-work, homelessness, and/or substance-use experience and have come from diverse corners of the trans communities in order to allow others to benefit from their experiences navigating social and health services. They must have all these qualifications, as well as a belief in the positive side of being a visible trans-person, having incorporated their current or past street-active experiences into their lives and proud identity. Instead of endlessly horrifying others with the dark side of sex work and drugs (which is a sure-fire self-esteem killer, not to mention a self-righteous position indicative of an elitist trans-politic), we maintain that these experiences can become part of a transsexual's proud life, as they are for many of us. We simply need information to be safe, healthy and happy. Here is how one peer support program was developed.

Early in 1998, Mirha-Soleil Ross was hired by the 519 Church Street Community Centre in Toronto to develop a community program for street-active transsexuals and transgender people. While there were support groups focusing on transition, many lower income and street-active trans people — especially youth — were finding it difficult to connect with people whose only barrier to being trans was transitioning. Many active trans groups also were not sex-worker positive, despite the fact that sex work is a vibrant part of transsexual women's culture and community.

A drop-in program, Meal Trans, was developed where people could come together socially while being able to get things they need. The primary need: a free healthy meal. Program development drew on models of peer support like CACTUS and ASTT(é)Q in Montreal, and based its design on interviews with as many lower-income and street-active trans people as possible. (See Bibliography on page 171 for addresses and telephone numbers for these support groups.)

Monica Forrester and I came on board in 1999 to do outreach to TS/TG sex workers in Toronto. The seroprevalence of HIV is very high with these women, and yet there were no services or outreach resources of any kind available to them. We consulted (and confirmed), asking what the women wanted, until we developed "The Happy Transsexual Hooker" — an HIV/AIDS information and prevention booklet that is quite possibly the first of its kind designed and produced entirely by TS/TG sex workers. The booklet was a huge hit, because *it was made by the people it was marketed for* — a basic tenant of all our peer-support programming.

Mirha-Soleil founded Meal Trans on a very special philosophy — that the program be directed by TS/TG people who have first hand experience with lower income, street-active and sex-worker experience, and that the participants who accessed the program always determined the direction of all activities and resources the program developed. With participation from our community we focused only on the urgent needs our participants brought to us. The participants are thought of as consultants to the programming we develop, such as our shelter and hostel staff training program, and Trans · Youth · Toronto!, a drop-in by and for TS/TG youth twenty-six years of age and under. We also work hard to empower all our participants by offering volunteer jobs (look at me, I started there as a volunteer), opportunities to train as peer mentors — who offer referrals, advocacy and a friendly ear to participants at the drop-in — and chances to train as workshop facilitators on issues of lower-income and street-active TS/TG people.

For any model of peer support, it is essential not to assume what the needs of the community you are serving are and drive ahead based on assessments performed by non-affected people. Meal Trans is proof that if you hire from the community with the mission to serve based on the needs of those you are working for, and get them involved in decisions that affect them, well then ... your success is almost always guaranteed.

Barriers that one must keep in mind are protecting your participants from exposure and staying rooted in the philosophy of peer support. This means being involved with media only as it benefits the participants, and never sending a volunteer or staff into a situation where they are targeted. It's important not to get discouraged if you consult with your participants on a new project and interest is very low. The need always comes from the community you serve, so never let your ego or hope for future plans get ahead of what everyone else needs and wants.

PEER SUPPORT, TRANSSEXUAL HEALTH & TRANSITIONING

Sadly, not a whole lot is known about the specifics of medical transsexual health. At the beginning of a transsexual's transition, it is more difficult to anticipate overall physical health in the years to come than it is to proactively decide current options. Options may include decisions about hormone replacement therapy (getting on testosterone or taking anti-testosterone drugs with estrogen), top surgeries (breast augmentation/reduction), bottom surgeries (surgical construction of a penis or vagina), facial surgeries (eyes, ears, nose, forehead, brow lifts, etc.), and facial hair removal (laser or electrolysis) — to name just a few. While it is very true that we may transition toward sexes, there are some physical things that we don't leave behind. I have simply come to call these matters "cross-over health concerns": health conditions we carry with us as we change our physical sex characteristics toward the sex we know we are.

Questions of transsexual health are numerous. Should transsexual men be getting Pap smears regularly? Should transsexual women be getting their prostates checked? What about breast cancer? What about testicular cancer? What about testicular cancer if you have no testicles but still have the testicular sac? I have already had one 'empty sac' exam (at my doctor's insistence) and the results were inconclusive. The primary answer to these questions is: if you think you should be checking it, then you probably should.

So why don't we look out for these health matters, especially when they might have the potential to make us very sick if unchecked? Maybe it's partly because we're afraid. No one wants to get sick, much less get sick with something associated with the sex we are transitioning away from. Maybe it's partly because our physicians stop thinking about our bodies as a whole and simply think of them as the sex that we are presenting. And, sadly, maybe it is because many physicians may have personal problems with our bodies and simply don't want to deal with it, even if they prescribe hormone replacement therapy. (Now if only we could get them to do actual research on hormones

themselves …) Peer support and community efforts allow these questions to come to the surface, to be discussed and thought about in a safe environment. They allow us to strategize steps and encourage informed, thoughtful decision-making. Creating such a safe environment takes into account that self-esteem and informed personal choice are paramount.

Sex reassignment surgeries are not a reality for most transpeople, as surgeries can cost from five thousand dollars well into tens of thousands of dollars. Top surgery, the lesser costing of these surgeries, may be a more likely surgery to be accessed. Peer support programming can assist people facing this physiological transition through surgery by sharing information about surgeons willing to perform the surgeries, what results others have had, and what risks are faced. The emotional responses pre- and post-surgery, as well as nitty-gritty hands-on post-surgical support may be found within a peer support model as well. The reality is that *basic* transition resources, such as hormone replacement, are difficult to access. And sex reassignment surgeries, assuming a transperson is financially able, are still at the stage where follow-up care is either discretionary, improvisational, or nonexistent. This is part of why peer support programming is essential.

None of this, however, compares to an even more dangerous trend with many physicians around the treatment of transsexuals. Epidemics such as HIV and hepatitis are ravaging our community, and despite the efforts of a few strong and loud community members, there has been little response globally from health services. Some reports peg the prevalence of HIV in transsexual sex-worker populations to be as high as 80 percent, making it the highest sero-prevalence of any marginalized community. And this community is not getting any specific treatment, mass outreach, or targeted care within the specific context of their sexuality, their bodies, and their lives. It seems like even the little things, such as possible reactions when taking both anti-AIDS medication and hormone replacement therapy, get missed. While studies show that there is probably very little interaction, one hormone — Estinyl — has been taken off the market since it was having a nasty side-effect when combined with anti-retroviral meds. It is apparent that this was known for years preceding the hormone's recall. What about lipodystrophy — changes of fat redistribution in the body and related irregularities in certain blood tests some people with HIV on anti-HIV therapy develop? Its true prevalence is unknown. What about health services that refuse to offer injectable estrogens to street-active populations even when individuals might be taking medication, be habitual substance users, and have hep-C? For TS/TG people, this is basic stuff. Naturopaths do say that the body's health system centres on the liver — and it is safe to say that your liver will be very stressed if you have many of these factors affecting your life and body. With all these questions, stigma over treatment remains the primary barrier for most people accessing street-active health services.

Rampant poverty is one of the biggest barriers to overcome within most of the TS/TG communities. We must work toward ending the stigma against prostitution and fighting for the decriminalization of sex work so that all prostitutes, escorts and strippers can work with more dignity, safety and greater financial stability. We must ensure that everyone has access to shelter and housing in a safe accessible environment. We must get people to recognize that substance users have rights too, and should be supported in their efforts to use drugs safely in a stigma-free environment. Finally, breaking down the prejudices that society at large has of those with physical disabilities and mental health issues is crucial. We should dismiss no one, but rather

go the extra mile to make workplaces and services accessible for all.

These barriers affect many marginalized communities, not just transpeople. A final goal is to unite and work with marginalized populations to fight racism, classism, poverty, homelessness, imperialism, ableism, homophobia, animal cruelty and transphobia, because we are all affected by these things. With us all united, the powers that be can never hope to stop us. There is another way to describe peer support — we can call it "community." However, there are many struggles and barriers within any given marginalized community. The trans-communities need desperately to support and validate their sex workers, homeless, substance users, youth, and transpeople of colour. In a way, most of our issues are many communities' pressing issues. To really support our peers, we have to recognize our own privilege and not be so quick to assume that others started out exactly where we did. Then we can truly hear each other's experiences as peers.

We are so worth it!

CHRISTINA STRANG has been a member of the trans communities in Toronto since she transitioned in her late teens. A woman of many lives, she is and has been: an artist, an activist, a film maker, an addict, a hooker, a community worker, a vegetarian, a goth and a proud transsexual woman. Recovering from years of substance use, she went on to develop The Happy Transsexual Hooker, Canada's first HIV/AIDS information and prevention campaign for transsexual and transgender sex workers. Christina is now the Community Partnership Coordinator with Voices of Positive Women, a provincial organization for HIV-positive women.

NUTRITION FOR BREAST HEALTH

Jen Green

The following dietary recommendations are appropriate for fibrocystic breast disease and breast cancer prevention, as well as general health and wellness. The idea is to cultivate a diet that is low in refined sugar and flour, low on the food chain, high in whole foods and rich in nutrients. Please note that the term "women" is used below where research has been done on women. Otherwise gender-neutral language is used to include FTM (female-to-male) guys.

FRUITS AND VEGETABLES

Aim to eat six to nine servings of fruit and vegetables per day; a serving equals one-half cup of cooked vegetables, one cup of salad or one large piece of fruit. This sounds like a lot of fruit and vegetables, but it ensures adequate vitamins, antioxidants and fibre, while leaving less room for junk food. Cancer fighting foods include:

- cabbage, broccoli, cauliflower, Brussels sprouts, kale, bok choy, kohlrabi, turnips (which all contain indoles and isothiocyanates)
- tomatoes, red grapefruit (rich in lycopene)
- spinach, collards (rich in lutein)
- garlic, onions, leeks (which contain allyl sulphides)
- parsley, carrots, kale, winter squash, apricots, cantaloupe, sweet potatoes (which contain allyl sulphides)
- red clover sprouts, broccoli sprouts and mung bean sprouts (rich in isoflavones)[1]

Antioxidants are essential nutrients found in fruit and vegetables. They decrease inflammation and protect DNA from the damage of free radicals, thereby reducing the risk of cancer and counteracting some of the effects of aging. Antioxidant supplements include vitamin A, vitamin C, vitamin E, CoQ10, selenium, turmeric, quercetin and green tea. Total antioxidant status reduces breast cancer risk[2] and cancer risk generally. Organic green tea is a wonderful antioxidant for cancer prevention, and may be especially helpful for women with breast cancer who are Her-2/neu positive.[3] You can drink two cups daily, unless you are sensitive to the caffeine it contains. If you have fibrocystic breasts, pay special attention to whether the green tea increases your breast tenderness and if this is the case, stop drinking it.

Turmeric, which contains curcumin, is a yellow spice that is extremely promising for fighting breast cancer. Curcumin prevents new blood vessel growth to tumours (anti-angiogenesis), is a powerful antioxidant, encourages liver detoxification, decreases inflammation, and has been shown to induce programmed cell death of cancer cells (apoptosis) in vitro.[4] Turmeric can be used liberally in cooking (one teaspoon daily) or taken as a supplement. Turmeric should be avoided during chemotherapy.[5,6] However, turmeric is safe for long-term use once conventional cancer treatments are over.

Shitake and maitake mushrooms are other foods that help to prevent cancer by boosting the immune system, especially natural killer cells. These medicinal mushrooms can be eaten liberally, especially around surgery, radiation and chemotherapy, when the immune system needs support.

Phytoestrogens

Phytoestrogens are plant chemicals that act like weak estrogen in the body. They are amphoteric, which means that if there is too much estrogen (which contributes to fibrocystic breast disease and breast cancer), they will block the estrogen receptor site. If there is not enough estrogen (such as in menopause), they will weakly activate the receptor site to help prevent osteoporosis. Types of phytoestrogen include genistein and daidzen (soya, miso, tofu, clover sprouts) and lignins (ground flaxseeds and pumpkin seeds).

Organic soya products are wonderful because they are antioxidants, make platelets less sticky, lower cholesterol, help liver detoxification, induce apoptosis, prevent cancer cells from multiplying, and inhibit blood vessels that feed cancer (anti-angiogenesis). In Asian countries, where breast cancer rates are at least two-thirds lower than in North America, the average soya consumption is thirty-five to sixty grams per day.[7] In a case controlled study of Asian–American women, women who ate soya at least once weekly during adolescence had a significantly reduced risk of breast cancer, and those who ate it during adult life showed a trend towards less breast cancer.[8] When increasing soya intake, include a source of iodine (seaweed, fish, iodized salt) to compensate for the way that soya reduces iodine uptake. Please note that if you are on tamoxifen, you should use soya only in moderation (one to three times weekly) and avoid genistein supplements until more research has been done. In laboratory studies, soya reduced tamoxifen's effectiveness,[9] while in animal studies it improved tamoxifen's effectiveness.[10] The scenario where soya is most seriously in question is in post-menopausal women with estrogen-positive tumors. What is desperately needed is research done on actual women with breast cancer who are consuming soya.

Ground flaxseeds are another incredible food for the breasts. They are an excellent source of fibre, phytoestrogens, and omega-3 fatty acids. Flaxseeds were shown to decrease tumour size between the time of diagnosis and the time of surgery in women with breast cancer who included it in their diet.[11] Grind two tablespoons of fresh flaxseeds daily and add them unheated over your cereal, salad or vegetables.

Another area requiring research is the effect of phytoestrogens on transgendered men and women. Phytoestrogens increase steroid-binding globulin levels, which are the transport system that carries hormones to their receptors. This could possibly decrease circulating hormone levels, or increase the way they bind to receptors. We just don't know. Either way, every person responds to hormone therapies in a unique way. Ideally, do a controlled experiment for a month. For FTM guys who still have a menstrual period, experiment to see if daily flaxseeds and soya increase or decrease menstrual symptoms. For MTF (male to female) women with breast tenderness, experiment with daily flaxseeds and soya and assess if it reduces pain. In both transgendered men and women, soya and ground flaxseeds are helpful in preventing heart disease, cancer and osteoporosis. If phytoestrogens don't seem to effect hormone therapies, they are a great idea to include in your diet for overall health and wellness.

Fats

In order to keep your breasts and heart healthy, fat should account for no more than 20 percent of your total caloric intake. However, don't be fooled into eating lots of "lite" and "low-fat" processed foods because they are usually loaded with sugar, which contributes to breast cancer.[12] Simply be selective about your fats. Use olive oil (two tablespoons daily) as your main cooking and dressing oil because it decreases the risk of breast cancer.[13]

Avoid all hydrogenated fats (fats that have trans-fatty acids in them). Hydrogenated fats are found in margarine, chips, fried food and many commercial baked goods. Minimize saturated fats, which are found in red meat, dairy, vegetable shortening, palm and coconut oil.[14]

It is vital to include essential fatty acids such as omega-3 and omega-6 fatty acids in your diet. These fats should be stored in the fridge and used unheated. Omega-6 oils to include in your diet are: raw nuts and seeds (almonds, sunflower seeds, sesame and pumpkin seeds) and evening primrose oil (especially if you have fibrocystic breast disease[15]). Evening primrose oil causes breast tissue to be less sensitive to estrogen and it offers a protective effect against breast cancer.[16] [17] Evening primrose oil also increases the effectiveness of tamoxifen in reducing estrogen-receptor expression.[18]

Omega-3 fatty acids to include in your diet are fish oils and walnuts. These oils decrease inflammation in the body, which makes them useful for treating conditions such as cancer, arthritis and eczema. They also make hair and nails grow stronger. High fish-oil intake is associated with lower rates of breast cancer.[19] The best fish oil to use is herring oil from Norway, because it is a smaller fish sourced from clean waters. This means it is less likely to accumulate toxins. Flaxseed oil, which is another omega-3 fatty acid, has recently become controversial in breast health. Ground flax seeds are undoubtedly good for breast cancer prevention. However, there is some evidence to suggest that flaxseed *oil* in very large amounts may encourage tumour growth.[20] Until more research is done, use a maximum of one teaspoon of flaxseed oil daily and consider herring oil instead.

Fibre

Women with a high-fibre diet have 30 percent less risk of breast cancer than women who have little fibre in their diets.[21] Fibre decreases cholesterol, regulates blood sugar, decreases estrogen and prevents colon cancer. Aim for thirty grams daily in the form of flax seeds, psyllium, wheat bran (if tolerated), legumes, fruit and vegetables.

For transgendered people, stay on a high-fibre diet while determining your ideal hormone levels. Be aware that fibre can decrease the absorption of many medications, including hormones. However, as long as your fibre intake is constant, you get the best of both worlds — action of the medication and healthy intestines.

Meat and Dairy

Meat and dairy products accumulate toxins as they move up the food chain and are therefore a major source of pesticides, hormones and antibiotics. The incidence of all types of cancer is 30 to 40 percent lower in Seventh Day Adventists, who are strict vegetarians.[22] Aim to have a primarily vegetarian diet with tofu, nuts and seeds, almond butter, and beans and rice. If you do not feel healthy on a protein-balanced vegetarian diet, eat organic meat and dairy in moderation, and fish from clean waters (if there is such a thing). Do not have large fish such as tuna, swordfish, mackerel or shark more than once a week to once a month, because they have toxic levels of mercury.[23]

Methylxanthines

Women with premenstrual breast tenderness should reduce or completely avoid substances containing methylxanthines. It is suggested that women with fibrocystic breast disease have a genetically determined sensitivity to methylxanthines.[24] Methylxanthines are found in coffee, black tea and chocolate.

Attitudes to Eating

All of us have some emotional issues around food. Whether we deprive ourselves, overeat to fill empty places, or eat destructively, diet is a loaded area for most people. Take time to be conscious of your eating patterns. Are you eating on the run so that your body has no chance to digest? Are you aware of hunger when you feel it? Are you aware of when you feel full? Is cooking for yourself part of your self-care? Try to have a gentle attitude with yourself around food choices. Too often, healthy foods can be associated with punishment and poor food choices symbolic of self-love. See if there can be some realignment, where the food that we know is healthy for us is perceived for what it really is … self-nurturing.

Conclusion

Nutrition is a way that we can be proactive about improving our health. We can support our breasts and our whole body by including phytoestrogens, fruits and vegetables, fibre and healthy fats in our diet. We can also minimize fried food, red meat, caffeinated drinks and junky food. See also the Bibliography in this book for additional resources.

Notes

1. Sat Dharam Kaur, *A Call to Women: The Healthy Breast Program and Workbook* (Kingston: Quarry Health Books, 2000), 193–229.
2. Ching, Ingram et al., "Serum levels of micronutrients, antioxidants and total antioxidant status predict risk of breast cancer in case control study," *Journal of Nutrition* (February 2002), 303–6.
3. Pianetti, Guo et al., "Green tea Polyphenol EGCG Inhibits Her-2/neu signalling, proliferation, and transformed phenotype of breast cancer cells," *Cancer Research* (February 2002), 652–5.
4. Choudhuri, Pal, et al., "Curcumin induces apoptosis in human breast cancer cells through dependent bax induction," *FEBS Letters* 512, nos. 1–3 (2002), 334–40.
5. I. Sriganth, et al., "Dietary curcumin with cisplatin administration modulates tumor market indices in experimental fibrosarcoma," *Pharmaceutical Research* 39 (1999), 175–9.
6. S. Somasundaram et al., "Dietary curcumin inhibits chemotherapy-induced apoptosis in models of human breast cancer," *Cancer Research* 62, no. 13 (July 2002), 3868–75.
7. Kaur, Ibid.
8. A.H. Wu, P. Wan et al., "Adolescent and adult soy intake and risk of breast cancer in Asian Americans," *Carcinogenesis* 23, no. 9 (September 2002), 1491–6.
9. Y.H. Ju et al., "Dietary Genistein Negates the Inhibitory Effect of Tamoxifen on Growth of Estrogen-dependent MCF-7 Cells Implanted in Athymic Mice," *Cancer Research* 62, no. 9 (May 2002), 2474–7.
10. A. Constantinou et al., "Consumption of soy products may enhance tamoxifen's breast cancer protective effects," *Proceedings of the American Association of Cancer Research* 42 (2001), 826.
11. Lilian Thompson, "Flaxseed and its lignin and oil components reduce mammary tumour growth at a late stage of carcinogenesis," *Carcinogenesis* 17, no. 6 (1996), 1373.
12. S. Austin, and C. Hitchcock, *Breast Cancer– What You Should Know (But May Not Be Told) About Prevention, Diagnosis and Treatment* (Rocklin: Prima, 1994), 167–89.
13. J. St. Martin-Moreno, W. Willett, L. Gorgojo et al., "Dietary fat, olive oil intake and breast cancer risk," *International Journal of Cancer* 58 (1994), 774–80.
14. Kaur, Ibid.
15. N. Pashby, "Clinical experience of drug treatment for mastalgia," *Lancet* 2 (1984), 373–7.
16. D. Horrobin, "Nutritional and medical importance of gamma-linolenic acid," *Progress in Lipid Research* 31 (1992), 163–94.
17. Tori Hudson, "Women's Health Update: Essential Fatty Acids and Breast Cancer," *Townsend Letter for Doctors & Patients*, 190 (May 1999), 129–32.
18. F. Kenny, S.E. Pinder, I.O. Ellis et al., "Gamma linolenic acid with tamoxifen as primary therapy in breast cancer," *International Journal of Cancer* 85 (2000), 643–8.
19. Hudson, Ibid.
20. Ibid.
21. T.E. Rohan et al., "Dietary fiber, vitamins A, C, E and the risk of breast cancer: a cohort study," Cancer Causes and Control (January 1993), 29–37; P.A. Baghurst, "High-fiber diets and reduced risk of breast cancer," *International Journal of Cancer* 56, no. 2 (January 1994), 173–6.
22. P.K. Mills, "Cancer incidence among Seventh-Day Adventists: 1976–1982," *American Journal of Clinical Nutrition* 59, no. 5 (suppl) (May 1994), 1136S–42S.
23. Health Canada, Mercury and Fish Consumption Advisory, www.cfia-aciaagr.ca/english/corpaffr/foodfacts/mercurye.html.
24. J. Minton et al., "Clinical and biochemical studies on methylxanthine–related FBD," *Surgery* 90 (1981), 229–304.

Naturopathic Approaches to Breast Surgery

Jen Green

What is Naturopathic Medicine?

Naturopathic medicine is a comprehensive system of health care combining conventional medical diagnosis with natural therapies. Naturopathic doctors are the general practitioners of complimentary and alternative medicine. They are trained to be primary health-care providers who offer nutrition, herbal medicine, homeopathy, lifestyle counselling, acupuncture and Chinese herbs. All of these therapies are aimed at treating the root causes of disease, supporting the body's innate ability to heal, and addressing the whole person. For a referral to a naturopathic doctor in your area, call the Ontario Association of Naturopathic Doctors at 1-877-628-7284. They can refer you to your provincial organization.

When you visit a licensed naturopathic doctor, you know that they have completed standardized North American examinations measuring their competency in subjects such as physical exam, pathology, laboratory and differential diagnosis. Your naturopathic doctor will refer you to conventional medical doctors whenever necessary. An initial visit typically lasts ninety minutes and will cover all aspects of your health history and present concerns. Feeling comfortable with and connected to your naturopathic doctor is an important part of the therapeutic relationship.

The health information presented in these sections is based on the current research, training and professional experience of the author, and is true and complete to the best of her knowledge. However, it is not intended to replace the advice given by the reader's personal physician or naturopathic doctor. Each person has a unique health situation, and should check with a qualified health-care professional for the appropriateness of supplements, herbs and exercise. The author and publisher are not responsible for any adverse effects or consequences resulting from the use of the information in this book. It is the responsibility of the reader to consult a qualified health-care professional. It is a sign of strength and wisdom to seek a second or third opinion.

Pre-Surgery Care

For starters, a healthy person makes a healthier surgery patient. This means taking time to eat a balanced diet, exercise, get fresh air and relax. Many people will stay busy before surgery to keep their minds occupied. However, pre-surgery can be a great opportunity to nurture yourself and stay present for what is happening.

Take time to visualize yourself going through the surgery. You may wish to let go of something symbolically if you are having your breast removed, or symbolically call something into your life if you are having breast enhancement or reconstruction.

Surgery can become a right of passage that takes on sacred and personal meaning for each individual. For example, one woman I work with painted a henna tattoo around her scar with her children to help reclaim her body.

You may also want to practise a particular relaxation, visualization or breathing exercise in advance so that just before the surgery you can use these same images. In a randomized study, patients who practised deep breathing and relaxation required 50 percent less post-operative narcotics, and were considered ready for discharge by their surgeons 2.7 days earlier than the control group.[1] Another study found that patients who practised relaxation had decreased post-operative pain, decreased narcotic use, decreased length of hospital stay, decreased post-operative blood pressure, heart rate and respiratory rate, and decreased anxiety.[2] Some ideas for visualization include imagining yourself in a special place, surrounding yourself with white light, and hanging your worries on a worry tree. Many different breathing exercises can be used from yoga or Qi Gong. I personally like to picture an ocean of healing filling up my lungs and washing me clean.

One to two weeks before surgery it is crucial to stop taking the following herbs and supplements, which can thin the blood and increase bleeding: vitamin E, vitamin C, gingko, feverfew, garlic, ginger, Asian ginseng and conventional blood-thinners. Continuing your regular multivitamin is fine, and actually advisable to maintain optimum nutritional status.

Note: If you are a pre-menopausal woman with breast cancer, schedule your mastectomy or lumpectomy in the second half of your menstrual cycle (luteal phase). A number of studies have shown that this can increase survival rates.[3] If you are someone who feels very connected to the moon, you may choose to avoid surgery on the full moon because some people believe there is more bleeding at this time.

Post-Surgery Care

Nutrition and Nutrients

People's digestive tracts are often sensitive after surgery, so plan ahead by preparing food that is nour-ishing and simple to absorb. Cook and freeze a number of soups to have brought to the hospital and/or to be eaten when you first get home. Try to include a protein source such as blended soft tofu, lentils, almond butter, egg drop, or organic chicken in each soup. Also use aromatic spices in the soups to aid digestion, for example ginger, garlic, cinnamon, clove, cardamom, thyme, fennel and anise. Preparing soup for you can be a great way for friends or family to show their support.

Post-surgery nutritional supplements can be very helpful in enhancing the body's wound repair. Consider a good quality multivitamin plus additional vitamin A, vitamin C, vitamin E and zinc. Often you can find a combination of A, C, E and zinc all in one. These vitamins have been shown to improve post-operative immune function and enhance wound healing.[4] Make sure to take the zinc with food, however, because it can cause nausea when taken on an empty stomach. If you have pre-existing digestive problems, choose a liquid or chewable multivitamin.

Nausea and Anaesthetics

If you experience nausea from the anaesthetic, you can drink grated ginger tea and wear a magnet or use acupressure on the acupuncture point PC6 (three finger widths/two inches above the inner wrist crease in the center of your arm between the two tendons).[5] A meta-analysis (collection of research) on acupuncture/acupressure for post-operative nausea and vomiting found that acupuncture/acupressure resulted in prevention equivalent to standard anti-nausea drugs.[6]

If you are spacey and disoriented after anaesthetic or craving cold and carbonated drinks, your naturopathic doctor may advise you to use homeopathic phosphorus 30CH; two pellets once daily for up to three days. If you are nauseous persistently, vomiting, or feel aggressive post-surgery, your naturopathic doctor may advise you to use homeopathic nux vomica/collubrina 30CH. All homeopathic pellets should be dissolved under the tongue away from food. Homeopathic remedies act as messages to the body asking the body to self-correct. Connect with a naturopathic doctor or experienced homeopath for more information on homeopathy.

Herbs can be taken after surgery to encourage liver detoxification and clear out the anaesthetic. Your naturopathic doctor or herbalist may advise you to use milk thistle in capsule or tincture form. Dosage is usually 150 to 200 mg capsules three times daily or sixty drops of tincture twice daily. Milk thistle is one of the few herbs that is better to take in capsule form because not all active constituents are water soluble. You may also find a good liver combination that includes herbs such as dandelion, beet root, artichoke or turmeric in addition to the milk thistle. Do not take liver herbs if you are dependent on medications that are effective only at a narrowly defined range (narrow therapeutic window), because the herbs can increase detoxification and clearance of medications. All herbs are best absorbed when taken away from food.

Wound Care

Follow the wound care directions given to you by your surgeon. Remember to change dressings as advised and keep the area clean. Once the incision site is closed superficially, you can use an herbal oil or salve topically to speed the rest of the wound repair. Salves that contain calendula, comfrey and St. John's wort are especially good. Calendula is a healing herb that can be made into a tea or used topically. It grows beautifully in the garden and is a blessing to watch flower.

To reduce bruising and swelling post-surgery, your naturopathic doctor may advise you to use homeopathic arnica 30CH. You can also use Traumeel homeopathic cream topically around the breast but not over the open wound. Bromelain, a naturally occurring pineapple enzyme, decreases bruising and post-operative pain.[7] Bromelain is a natural anti-inflammatory that is a good alternative to non-steroidal anti-inflammatory drugs because it does not cause digestive upset. It reduces post-surgical swelling and has proven effective in a double-blind crossover trial.[8] There has been concern about the anticoagulant effects of bromelain. However, while bromelain acted as a blood-thinner in animal studies, human research fails to show that it thins the blood in any clinically significant way.[9] Additionally, bromelain has anti-tumour activity and stimulates immune responses in breast cancer patients.[10] A typical dose is 500 to 750 mg three times daily away from food.

If pain persists after the first few days after surgery, consider a homeopathic. If the chest feels bruised or achey after three days, your naturopathic doctor may advise you to take homeopathic bellis perennis 30CH twice daily for two days. If there are shooting pains, numbness or tingling after surgery and you are forgetful, blue or sensitive to touch, you may be advised to use hypericum 30CH. If the pain is out of proportion to the surgery, you may be advised to use calendula 30CH. If you have stitching pains, are hypersensitive to touch and feel violated by the surgery, staphysagria 30CH may be recommended. See a naturopathic doctor for more detailed prescriptions or if pain persists more than a few weeks after surgery.

Lymphatic Drainage

Often after surgery there is lymphatic swelling/lymphedema because the normal pathways of drainage have been disrupted. This can happen especially if lymph nodes have been removed or if there is extensive scar tissue. Mechanical therapies such as dry skin brushing, lymphatic massage, and arm exercises help with circulation. (See also the chapter in this book on lymphatic drainage.) Additionally, herbs can be used to reduce swelling and increase lymphatic flow. These include burdock, calendula, goldenseal, red root, phytolacca, red clover, cleavers, wild indigo, scrophularia, stillingia and iris versicolour. Pre-mixed tinctures such as Hoxsey Formula (many brands), the Healthy Breast Formula (St. Francis), Cleaver's Combo (St. Francis) or custom-made formulas can be used. Herbs are natural drugs, so see a qualified practitioner for doses and a combination that best suits you. If there are no qualified practitioners in your area, drink a pot of tea made from red clover, Cleaver's and calendula daily.

The final and most essential naturopathic aspect of surgical care is the inner faith and knowledge that your body can heal. I have been lucky to work with many people who have deep trust in their bodies. I am reminded that an important part of my work is simply to witness the incredible healing power of nature!

JEN GREEN completed a Bachelor of Arts and Science at McMaster University before becoming a Doctor of Naturopathic Medicine. She helped to initiate a breast cancer prevention and treatment program at the Canadian College of Naturopathic Medicine, where she lectures regularly on women's health and breast cancer. Jen served as the Vice President of the Canadian Naturopathic Association and received an award for clinical excellence in the naturopathic treatment of women's health. Jen is in private practice in downtown Toronto.

NOTES

1. Judith J. Petry, "Surgery and Complimentary Therapies: A Review," *Alternative Therapies in Health & Medicine* 6, no. 5 (September, 2000), 64–74.
2. Ibid.
3. Susan Love, *Dr. Susan Love's Breast Book* (Third Edition. New York: Perseus, 2000), 376.
4. Petry, Ibid.
5. S.L. Dibble et al, "Acupressure for nausea — results of a pilot study," *Oncology Nursing Forum* 27 (2000), 41–7.
6. A. Lee, M.L. Done, "The use of nonpharmacologic techniques to prevent post-operative nausea and vomiting: a meta-analysis," *Anesthetic Analogue* 88 (1999), 1362–9.
7. Petry, Ibid.
8. G. Tassman et al., "A double-blind crossover study of plant proteolytic enzyme in oral surgery," *Journal of Dental Medicine* 20 (1965), 51–4.
9. J.E. Harris, "Interaction of dietary factors with oral anticoagulants: review and applications," *Journal of American Dietician Association* 95 (1995), 580–4.
10. K. Eckert et al., "Effects of oral bromelain administration on the impaired immunocytotoxicity of mononuclear cells from mammary tumor patients," *Oncology Report* 6 (1999), 1191–9.

Pre- and Post-Operative Care Through Traditional Chinese Medicine

Mary Wong

Traditional Chinese medicine (TCM) represents the oldest and most comprehensive system of health care in the world. This empirical science has developed over five thousand years, and is still used today as a primary system of health care in China alongside mainstream medicine. Although relatively new in the West, TCM is rapidly gaining acceptance as a safe and effective alternative or adjunct to western medicine. TCM is a time-honoured system of medicine involving the use of one or more treatments such as acupuncture, Chinese herbal medicine, Tui Na massage, exercise (Tai Chi, or Qi Gong), and dietary therapy.

The goal of the disciplines of Chinese medicine is to reestablish balance and order in the body, mind and spirit. The premise is to maintain health and longevity through prevention of illness. Although the focus is on prevention, TCM treats a variety of medical conditions.

In principle, the foundation of achieving and maintaining good health is through diet, exercise, adequate rest and relaxation, and a good mental attitude. In practice, however, changes in diet and lifestyle are often not enough to maintain good health in our high-stress, fast-paced society. During certain points in our lives, interventions such as acupuncture and herbal medicine may be a good alternative/adjunct to help us achieve optimal health. A similar analogy is car maintenance. If we use the appropriate gasoline, get regular oil changes and tune-ups, and drive responsibly, we can increase the lifespan of a car. However, without proper maintenance and care, the car would run into trouble very quickly. Unfortunately, most people tend to take better care of their cars than they do of themselves.

In the case of breast and chest surgery, Chinese medicine can be used to aid a smooth and healthy recovery pre- and post-operatively. To be specific, acupuncture and Chinese herbal medicine can help you strengthen yourself physically, mentally and emotionally before and after the surgery. Before looking at how TCM can help pre- and post-operative care, we must understand how this tradition's approach to health and well-being works.

TCM stems from a Taoist philosophy and has a holistic view of the body, mind and spirit. The Chinese believe that good health depends on the smooth flow of a vital energy, qi (pronounced "chee"), through the body. Qi is an all-pervasive energy that animates life and sustains everything around us. There are many manifestations of qi, from the very ethereal to the very physical, which, if it runs smoothly in our bodies, provides optimal health. This qi flows through a system of channels, like rivers and tributaries, that supply the entire body. If these energy channels flow smoothly, health flourishes. If there are blocks in any of these electrical pathways, over a period of time health may be compromised and disease may ensue.

In Chinese medical theory, there are internal and external causes for energy disruption. It is normal to experience emotions such as anger, joy, worry, sorrow and fear, but if one emotion predominates over others for prolonged periods and interferes with the conduct of daily life, then the smooth flow of qi may be disrupted. This causes an internally created climate for illness. External causes of disharmony relate to the external pernicious influences, for example climatic conditions such as wind, fire, heat, dryness, dampness and cold. For example, living in a cold damp basement apartment over a long period of time can cause arthritis or joints to stiffen and swell as the damp and cold invades the body and impedes blood flow. Other external miscellaneous factors include lifestyle, exercise, diet, work, sexual activity, constitution and trauma. Surgical procedures of any kind, including reduction, augmentation and mastectomy, are viewed as an assault on the body and may potentially become an external factor of illness. Incisions and transplants impede the flow of qi and blood in the network of vessels in the body. If the incisions do not heal properly, they can be an underlying cause for complications and illness. To be specific, blood can potentially accumulate and over time become stagnant. Water can also accumulate, which can cause the swelling or edema seen in breast cancer surgery (typically with edematous swelling of the upper arm). Swelling may eventually go away, but through Chinese medical intervention, healing may be augmented.

Acupuncture, Tui Na, herbal medicine, Tai Chi and Qi Gong are all modalities of Chinese medicine which aim to manipulate the channels of energy to regulate all physical and mental processes. Acupuncture, one of the most renowned components of TCM, involves the insertion of fine, disposable, pre-sterilized needles at specific locations along channels of the body where the qi can be influenced. They are not inserted into blood vessels or nerves, so, generally, there's no bleeding or pain involved. These meridians are invisible but exist under the skin and above the muscles where the tissues are most active electrically. They connect to the body's tissues and organs, and are manipulated through over 360 places identified as acupuncture points along the surface of the skin. There are fourteen main meridians, twelve of which take the names of their corresponding internal organs, such as the heart, liver, lungs, small intestines, etc. By stimulating the acupuncture points, the balance and flow of qi to the meridians and the associated organs is restored. Once the body's homeostasis is reestablished, the pathological condition is alleviated. According to the Chinese, disease is a pathological imbalance of energy, blood or fluids in the body's internal organs or channels. The insertion of needles or other stimulation at acupuncture points helps rebalance the body's energy.

An explanation proposed by Western scientists is that acupuncture may trigger the release of substances within the body called endorphins, which not only have a painkilling effect but also influence the whole autonomic nervous system. It may also alter the body's output of neurotransmitters such as serotonin and norepinephrine, and of inflammation-causing substances such as prostaglandins.

Note that whether one is on pharmaceutical medications or hormones for those who are transitioning, acupuncture provides a safe way of treatment without any negative interactions.

As mentioned previously, breast and chest surgery is considered to be a physical and emotional trauma to the body. Acupuncture treatments reestablish balance in the body by bolstering the qi, moving the blood, inhibiting water accumulation, dispersing swelling, opening the energy network vessels, and transforming stasis on a physical level. When acupuncture is used in combination with herbal medicine, the treatments become intensified, and healing may be augmented two-fold. Treatments may differ from one person to the next, because each person is individual and unique. Both of these healing modalities are powerful and should be taken only under the supervision of a trained professional.

Pre-Operative Care

To prepare for any surgery, one should be strong both physically and mentally. In terms of Chinese medicine, both acupuncture and Chinese herbal preparations can be used to maintain good flow of blood and energy throughout the body. The stomach channel in particular is directly associated to the breasts and breast tissues. As seen in the chart below, the meridian crosses directly over the breasts. Moreover, the stomach organ (together with the spleen), from the Chinese perspective, is considered to be the source of acquired energy through the nutrients from food and drink. Through acupuncture, we can strengthen the stomach organ by choosing points along the stomach energy pathway. Another very important organ related to the breasts is the liver, even though its related meridian doesn't traverse the breasts directly. The liver is in charge of promoting the smooth flow of qi energy and blood throughout the whole body. If this flow is impeded, then the energy and blood circulation to the breasts can be affected. So acupuncture may be used to open the flow to the breast via the liver.

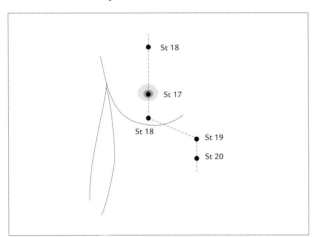

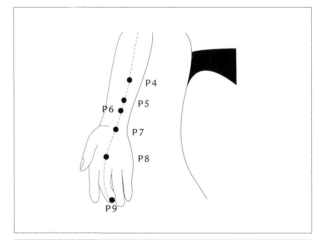

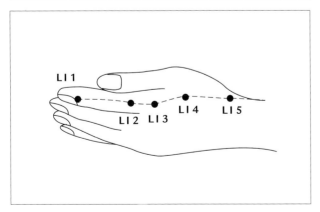

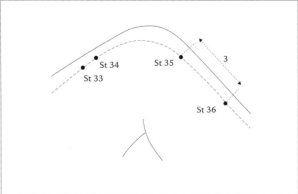

Pre-surgical anxiety is very common. Acupuncture can be used to ease the mind and induce restful sleep before surgery. Other things to do at home prior to surgery include meditation, yoga or Tai Chi for energy balance and stress reduction.

If there are other health concerns, such as generalized pain, a common cold or digestive discomforts, they should be addressed to minimize the stress of surgery. A good healthy diet is also important as a building block for health and recovery after surgery. Because each individual is made up differently, a detailed diet would be very difficult to recommend. Generally speaking, however, foods are categorized by nature. So, one living in a warm climate can get away with eating more "cooling" types of foods such as cucumber and watermelon. However, if one lives in a cold climate or season, you should consider drinking more warm fluids, eating warm foods, and using spices like ginger or clove. (For more specific information on diet, I would recommend *The Tao of Healthy Eating: Dietary Wisdom According to Chinese Medicine,* by Bob Flaws.)

POST-OPERATIVE CARE

As mentioned earlier, Chinese medicine can augment the rate of healing. Acupuncture can be used to stop pain and nausea and alleviate constipation and bloating, all of which are common post-surgical symptoms. Again, the meridian of choice would be through the stomach pathway. For healing of the site of incision, some needles can be inserted near but not directly into the scars. By increasing blood circulation to the local area, dispersing the accumulation of fluids, and decreasing inflammation, acupuncture and herbs will help to minimize pain and scarring both internally and externally.

Acupuncture can also have a profound effect on mood. Chinese medicine can tap into the autonomic nervous system and address mood changes such as post-surgical depression on a mental/emotional level. It can lift and the calm the spirit by promoting a smooth qi flow.

From the Chinese medical perspective, it is important to stay away from shellfish, greasy and spicy foods, alcohol, and cigarette smoking after surgery, since they are considered toxic and can complicate healing. Drinking plenty of water is beneficial to help flush out the body post-surgically.

Self-massage is another adjunct to healing. There are certain points that one can massage which affect the breast tissue area. Once the point is located, press your thumb on the point in a small circular fashion without lifting it off the point of contact. Stimulation of the point occurs when you feel a dull ache upon massaging. Press for several minutes. These points are based on the acupuncture points, which follow the meridian/energy pathways of the body. Since the stomach is the primary channel that runs through or around the breasts, it is recommended to find points along that channel to affect the breast/chest and breast tissues.

RECOMMENDED ACUPRESSURE POINTS

A point of advice is to find a practitioner first to show you how you can effectively utilize these techniques so that you can help yourself at home. However, you can refer to the chart included in this chapter to help you find the following points.

For breast/chest healing: The point St 18 Ru Gen (translated as "Breast's Root") is located directly under the nipple line between the fifth and sixth ribs bilaterally which is a local point for the breasts and chest. Then press St 36 Zu San li (or "Three Leg Miles"), which is a point one finger-width lateral to the tibia and about three units below the kneecap. This point will help direct qi and blood flow to aid healing.

For pain relief: Li 4 He Gu (or "Adjoining Valley"), which is the name of a famous acupuncture point located in the web of the hand between the thumb and index finger and can be massaged deeply to relieve pain affecting the area of the body from the diaphragm upwards. We can use this point to control pain post-surgically. To be effective, one must pinch and grasp the fleshy bit of skin closest to where the junction of the bones of the thumb and index finger meet and put enough pressure to cause a deep ache or bruising sensation, called Da Chi ("Grasping/hitting" the energy).

For nausea: Another useful point to locate is PC 6 Nei Guan ("Inner Gate"), approximately two inches above the wrist bone between the two tendons on the palmar aspect of the body. Again, one should press on the point to induce a dull ache if there is any sign of nausea.

To calm the mind: Use a knuckle and rub the point halfway between the inside edges of the eyebrows. This point is an extra point called Yin Tang ("Seal Hall").

Choosing an Acupuncturist

In most provinces, unfortunately, acupuncturists are not regulated. This means attention to detail is important in choosing your practitioner. Like specialists, one should look for a Doctor of Traditional Chinese Medicine, and not what I consider a "cookbook acupuncturist." There are short courses designed for professionals such as MDs and physiotherapists out there, but their knowledge of Chinese medicine tends to be limited. A Traditional Doctor has a minimum of three years full-time training. Diagnosis involves asking questions, looking at the tongue and feeling the radial pulse at the wrists. One source would be to get a list of practitioners from local regulating bodies for acupuncture. American states, however, do generally have licensing regulations for acupuncturists and practitioners of Chinese medicine. If your state has licensing laws, be sure that your acupuncturist has a current license with the state.

Mary Wong graduated with a B.Sc. in Biology at McMaster University and then went on to study at the Canadian College of Acupuncture and Oriental Medicine and graduated in 1993. She is a member of the Ontario Acupuncture Examination Committee and Ontario Association of Acupuncture and Traditional Chinese Medicine. She has lectured at such institutions as the Mount Sinai Hospital and the Canadian Breast Cancer Society. She has also been featured in the Alternative Health section of the NOW Magazine and has made a guest appearance on TV Ontario. Currently she is in private practice.

Swedish Massage

Sarah Cowley

Swedish massage given by a Registered Massage Therapist is legislated by the Regulated Healthcare Professionals Act, the governing body for doctors, nurses and physiotherapists, among others. Massage therapists are trained, educated professionals with yearly registration requirements. This registration provides therapists with a code of ethics and a standard of practice to work within as outlined by the College of Massage Therapists. A Registered Massage Therapist may continue with postgraduate education in specialized fields of therapy such as breast massage, hydrotherapy and manual lymphatic drainage. In Ontario, massage therapy has evolved into a medically oriented therapy where massage therapists consult and work in conjunction with other health-care professionals to provide a realm of optimal health and well-being for their clients.[1]

Massage therapy for breast health, breast or chest surgery, and sexual transitioning requires that a therapist have additional academic and technical training which includes a focus on relationship skills. This training ensures that individuals seeking therapy receive safe treatment, and that their needs and objectives for breast or chest surgery and medical alterations are understood by their therapist. It is important that you find a therapist with whom you can develop a trusting and safe relationship. This relationship must nurture a sense of well-being, and offer support for emotional as well as physical changes. For example, transsexual persons undergoing surgery as a part of transitioning will want a therapist who is attentive to the changing dynamics and levels of comfort with their chest/breast area as their identifying gender changes. The therapist's sensitivity to changing needs in the use of names, pronouns, and types or areas of touch is important.

(Please note that in this article, the terms "breast health" and "breast massage" are used to indicate both breast and chest health/massage.)

Pre-Operative

When you have chosen surgery such as gynaecomastia correction, augmentation, reduction or reconstruction as a treatment to meet your personal and medical needs, you may also consider breast massage as a treatment of choice for pre-operative care. Breast massage will improve the health of breast tissue and associated muscles by enhancing blood circulation and lymphatic drainage, eliminating impurities and promoting blood flow to reduce tissue congestion and tenderness.[2] However, breast massage is not recommended pre-operatively for an individual with breast cancer who has not received treatment for the cancer. Direct pressure or manipulation of a tumour could promote a release of malignant cells into blood and lymph circulation.[3]

Post-Operative

Post-operatively, breast massage is an appropriate therapy for breast surgery related to cancer and other surgeries. There are, however, special considerations to be aware of following surgery for the treatment of cancer which are detailed below. Post-operatively, massage therapy supports and enhances the body's blood and lymph systems to reduce tissue swelling and to provide an environment for optimal tissue healing and scar formation. Supporting tissue healing and scar formation may prevent pain and restrictions in the range of motion in the shoulder and torso.

Because massage enhances a body's blood and lymph flow, this treatment could influence metastasis of cancerous cells and cells that may have been released into the body's circulation during surgery. The environment of blood and lymph is hostile to cancerous cells because of the flow, so enhancement of these systems "may be as likely to jeopardize cell survival as support it."[4] As well, cancer and cancer therapies such as radiation and chemotherapy compromise the immune system and therefore may suppress physical wellness and the quality of healing. Healing of the incision may take longer, and there is a greater possibility of post-surgical infection.

A massage therapist must be aware of the signs and symptoms of delayed healing that could be detrimental. These signs and symptoms include changes in the experience of pain, inflammation of the surgical sites and surrounding tissue, and changes in body temperature systemically and locally at the affected sites. (These signs and systems apply to all surgeries.) These symptoms must be reported to the medical professionals caring for the client. The controversies already mentioned above regarding massage and possible metastasis must be discussed between the client and massage therapist before treatments begin. If massage is chosen to be part of a treatment plan soon after surgery then "consultation with the surgeon or oncologist is essential in order to weigh the advantages and disadvantages of early massage intervention."[5]

MAKING A DECISION

When breast massage therapy is considered a treatment of choice, discuss the reasons for your decision with your massage therapist to ensure you're clear about treatment and satisfied with the outcome of the treatment. As already mentioned, breast massage enhances circulation of blood and lymph to eliminate impurities, reduces tissue swelling and congestion, and acts as a preventative approach in maintaining healthy breast tissue.

When breast massage is not an appropriate therapy, you may choose a general massage for relief of anxiety and physical discomfort. Massage may encourage relaxation, which will enhance physical and emotional health and well-being.

Always discuss the possibility of self treatment with your physician and/or Registered Massage Therapist prior to commencing self breast massage or scar tissue massage.

SELF BREAST MASSAGE

You may wish to include self breast massage as a health and wellness self-care exercise. Share this information with the massage therapist and the physician prior to commencing. Self breast massage is a way of getting to know your breast without the anxiety or fear that often goes along with touching a breast for examination. Self breast massage is a time where you can touch and feel your breasts in a nurturing fashion to discover what normal breast tissue is for you and to recognize the changes that are taking place with involution and with medical intervention.

Generally speaking, self breast massage is a series of relatively easy techniques applied to the breast tissue. Begin by placing your hands on your breasts, covering your breast with your open hand. A gentle jiggle of the breast tissue combined with a gentle lifting and pulling away motion of the breast from the chest wall assists greatly with tissue drainage. With soft flat fingers, make small circles going round and round in larger circles, covering the entire breast including the armpit region. Use a blend of oils made especially for breast massage or use a cooking oil such as olive oil to avoid a tugging or friction on the skin. Use enough pressure so that you feel the underlying structures without causing physical discomfort. Self breast massage may also be done in the shower, in which case soap can be used to avoid tugging. Self breast massage can be a special time for reflection and relaxation.

Scar Tissue Massage

Massage for breasts with scar tissue is beneficial when the scar tissue is causing pain and pulling of surrounding tissue. Scar tissue may also cause a reduced range of motion of the shoulder or torso. Scar tissue may also hinder drainage of the breast region postoperatively. If pain and a reduction of movement occurs long after surgery, massage to the scar tissue is a possible therapy. A massage therapist would most likely include hydrotherapy and manual lymphatic drainage in the treatment to soften the scar tissue before applying specific massage techniques to release the fibrosed tissues in the scar. (See the individual chapters in this book on these techniques.) The massage treatments will vary depending on how soon after surgery they begin, the type of procedures performed, and how well you are feeling. Again, if the scarring is a result of cancer surgery there is a "risk of dislodging metastasizing cells. Consultation with the oncologist or current family practitioner should occur."[6] With guidance from your therapist, you may choose to support these treatments with self breast massage at home.

NOTES

1. F. Rattray, *Massage Therapy* (Toronto: Massage Therapy Texts and MAVerick Consultants, 1995).

2. Sat Dharam Kaur, *A Call to Women: The Healthy Breast Program and Workbook* (Kingston: Quarry Health Books, 2000).

3. Debra Curties, R.M.T., *Massage Therapy and Cancer* (Toronto: Sutherland-Chan Publications, 1998).

4. Ibid., 16.

5. Ibid., 19.

6. Ibid., 20.

Sarah Cowley is a Registered Nurse, a Registered Massage Therapist and a Certified Manual Lymph Drainage Therapist. She is currently working full time in her private practice in a small community northeast of Toronto providing massage therapy and manual lymph drainage to her clients. She teaches supporting breast health on a casual basis.

Hydrotherapy Massage

Gail Hancock

Massage therapists are also trained in hydrotherapy. Hydrotherapy is the use of water in any of its three forms — solid, liquid or vapour — and at various temperatures, such as ice, baths or steam respectively. The water can be taken internally or externally, either for the treatment of disease or trauma, or to maintain optimum health. Hydrotherapy treatments enhance blood and lymphatic circulation through the entire body. This increase in circulation results in more oxygen and nutrients being delivered to the tissues and an increase in the elimination of waste products (carbon dioxide by the lungs and metabolic wastes by the liver and kidneys) from the body.

One of the wonderful things about hydrotherapy is that water is free (well relatively!) and readily available to anyone who has a tap in their home. As well, many of the techniques used in hydrotherapy require no fancy equipment and are easily taught to patients, who can then do the treatments at home. This not only empowers patients, it also relieves you of the financial burden that doing a series of professional hydrotherapy treatments may bring. A word of caution: if you live in an older home you may have lead in your pipes. The water that remains overnight in such pipes may contain lead. In order to get fresh, uncontaminated water, you will need to flush this water out of the pipes. To do this, run the cold water tap in your bathroom and kitchen for a few minutes. It is a good idea

to do this again if you have been out of the house for a few hours. Also, never use hot tap water for any hydrotherapy treatment, as hot water will pull more lead from the pipes than cold. It is best always to start with cold water and heat it to the desired temperature.

When you present at your massage therapist's practice and advise that you are going to have surgery, the therapist will want to help you be as ready for the procedure as possible. While it is important for you to relax before surgery, the therapist will also aim to support your entire body by helping to improve overall circulation. This is where certain hydrotherapy techniques can be of benefit. Most of these in-office hydrotherapy techniques can be used both pre- and post-operatively, but the length and frequency of treatment will be adjusted to accommodate your needs. Post-surgery the treatments may be shorter and a little less often until you regain your health and vitality. When preparing for any type of hydrotherapy treatment, the therapist will take into account your mental, physical and emotional state. The therapist will also stay with you during the treatment to monitor any changes in pulse rate, colour and comfort level. If there is any type of negative reaction during the treatment, the treatment will be stopped. If there is a negative reaction after the treatment, the therapist will have to reassess and modify the treatment before administering it again. Symptoms of negative reactions are dizziness, headaches, palpitations, insomnia, hyperventilation, fainting, nausea and skin sensitivity. Overall, hydrotherapy can be used safely and effectively for everyone, but every patient is different. After taking a proper case history, the therapist may decide in some cases that certain medical conditions disallow such treatment.

In-Office Treatments

WET SHEET WRAP: A wet sheet wrap can be beneficial before surgery. This involves wrapping the entire body in a cold wet sheet with a wrapping of a number of dry blankets on the outside for anywhere from twenty minutes to two hours. Although it may sound uninviting, the procedure is actually a warming treatment and helps your circulation and overall metabolism by having the body react to the cold of the sheet. The therapist would adjust the duration of the treatment to achieve an appropriate outcome, to maximize relaxation, and to enhance circulation.

NEUTRAL BATH: Another pre-surgery treatment your therapist may suggest is a neutral bath, wherein you are immersed in bath water of approximately 36 to 37 degrees Celsius for fifteen minutes to one hour. The bath water is maintained at this temperature. It is a very good treatment for anxiety and insomnia.

HOT/COLD PACKS: For post-surgery techniques, ice packs applied locally for two to eight minutes can be used to decrease swelling, inflammation and pain. Once this goal has been achieved, a contrast hot pack and cold pack can be utilized to help increase circulation in the area directly affected by surgery.

SALT GLOWS: A salt glow is an application of wet salt that is rubbed briskly on the skin. The therapist uses approximately one kilogram of Epsom salts or pickling salt that has been moistened and applies it to the skin with back-and-forth friction until the skin turns pink. The skin is then rinsed and dried vigorously. This increases circulation, eliminates toxins through the skin and generally tones the body. Once again, this treatment can help a patient both pre- and post-surgery.

STEAM BATH: You are seated on a chair in a steam cabinet with your head outside the cabinet. The steam treatment lasts approximately five to ten minutes for a stimulating effect and fifteen to twenty minutes for a sedative effect. After the treatment you will be asked to take a short cold shower. This is very helpful for detoxifying the body, which may help after surgery to ease the "hangover" effect from any anaesthesia.

POULTICE: A poultice can help heal tissues affected by surgery. See "At-Home Treatments" below for details.

With all of these treatments the therapist will have you rest for twenty to thirty minutes afterwards. It is advisable to wait a week to ten days post-surgery before performing any hydrotherapy treatment directly on the site of the incision. This time will allow for the tissue to begin to repair. "Water can equalize the circulation of the blood, control and equalize temperature, relieve pain, stimulate a sluggish or inactive organ, remove foreign or toxic material from the system and stimulate or soothe the entire nervous system."[1] Because it works on the circulation (blood flow and lymphatic flow), we can manipulate our treatment or choose a treatment that will promote health and vitality to the body both pre- and post-surgery.

At-Home Treatments

DRY BRUSHING: One of the simplest treatments to do at home is dry brushing to the skin. The skin has many functions: external support of the body, regulation of body temperature, protection and elimination of waste materials. The dry brushing technique not only stimulates circulation, it also rids the skin of dead cells. This keeps the skin clean, thereby allowing it to deal efficiently with any waste material or toxins. This elimination process happens through the pores via perspiration. We can see that if the pores are clogged with dead skin cells, their function will be impeded, which means that waste material then has to be dealt with by other organs of elimination. This puts unnecessary stress on those organs. The technique itself is very simple.

Purchase a natural bristle brush or loofah with a handle, which will allow you to reach your back. Natural bristle brushes are of animal origin, while loofah is of plant origin — avoid nylon bristle brushes because of their synthetic nature. Both the natural brush and the loofah are widely available in drugstores, health food stores, etc. The last brush I purchased came from my local dollar store and cost me $3.00. The brushing should be gentle and should be done with small circular movements or long strokes, and towards the heart when possible. Standing in your bathtub start brushing from the feet upward. Your feet should be warm to start with. If they aren't, run them under some hot water until they feel warm.

Begin with your feet, then your legs, then your abdomen. Brush clockwise. Proceed to your chest, avoiding going over the nipples, then your arms. Finish with your back. The whole procedure should take about five minutes or so. It is best to do in the morning right before you take your shower. Once you have finished you should take a hot shower to remove all those dead cells. Continue with your regular showering routine, but at the end turn the shower to a cooler temperature and end the treatment this way. Allow your brush or loofah to dry between brushings. It is recommended that this technique be used only every second or third day to prevent the body from becoming dependent on this stimulus.

There are some circumstances in which dry brushing is not recommended. If you have a condition like eczema, which causes skin lesions, you should avoid the affected area and brush around it. If you have a condition like Cushing's syndrome, which causes easily broken skin, you should not do dry brushing treatments at all.

POULTICE: The poultice is a very old and effective treatment. It promotes wound healing and can decrease pain, swelling, congestion and inflammation. A poultice also helps prevent sepsis of incisions or wounds by curbing the growth of harmful microorganisms. If you are seeking hydrotherapy post-surgery, your therapist will want to consult with your surgeon or primary nurse to discuss a treatment plan for you. This enables your therapist to revise or modify the treatment to be of the most benefit to you and keeps the doctor advised of the situation.

A poultice is made up of a combination of clay, vegetables, herbs or castor oil, which is placed on the skin and covered with a cloth to keep it in place. Shredded vegetables (potatoes, carrots) and vegetable leaves (cabbage) are helpful in absorbing toxins from the incision site. Two herbs that are useful in healing are comfrey and calendula. You can use either the fresh herb (preferably) or the dried. The amount of material that you use will depend upon the area that you need to cover. The herbs should be boiled until they become mushy, then strained and pulverized in a food processor. They can either be applied directly onto the affected area or placed between layers of cheesecloth and then placed on the area. Shredded vegetables may also be applied directly or with cheesecloth. With cabbage, use a couple of large leaves, cut out the rib and press them under a glass bottle or rolling pin until the leaf turns a bit shiny (you are in effect breaking the inside of the leaf down which allows for the leaves to be of the most benefit). You can then place the cabbage leaves directly on the breast that you want to treat — since the leaves are somewhat curved they are a good fit for this area of the body.

With all of the above substances, you then wrap the area with a clean flannel or cotton sheet which has been folded into quarters lengthwise and then wrap this around the chest, from under the axilla. The wrapping should be secure but not too tight. Fasten the material with a bandage, tape or a safety pin and leave on for forty minutes to an hour. When done, throw out the plant or vegetable matter and launder your sheet. You can poultice daily to facilitate healing.

The poultice procedure is not recommended if you have an allergy to any of the poultice materials.

Water has spoken to people through the centuries when they were looking for healing techniques. It is sometimes an overlooked application because it seems too simple or accessible. However, it is a very gentle therapy which is non-invasive and seems to resonate well with our watery bodies. Trying one of these techniques will convince you of its effectiveness.

NOTE

1. Dian Dincin Buchman, *The Complete Book of Water Therapy* (New Canaan, Connecticut: Keats Publishing, Inc., 1994).

GAIL HANCOCK has been a registered massage therapist for eighteen years and is currently in private practice in Toronto. Her specialty is working with special needs clients. She is a teaching assistant in both the Hydrotherapy and Soft Tissue Manipulation programs at the Canadian College of Naturopathic Medicine and also has a special affinity for herbs.

LYMPHATIC DRAINAGE MASSAGE

Pam Hammond

Lymphatic drainage is a type of specialized, gentle massage used to facilitate lymph circulation. A certified lymph drainage therapist must successfully complete all levels of postgraduate training in combined decongestive therapy (lymph drainage, skin care and compression bandaging).

The lymphatic system is a delicate but strong network of lymph vessels, lymph nodes and lymphoid organs designed to protect us from disease. Lymph is a pale fluid resembling blood plasma found within the lymphatic vessels. It usually contains white blood cells but not red blood cells. Lymph is collected from tissues in all parts of the body and is filtered by the lymph nodes before it is returned to the heart via the lymphatic ducts. Its purpose is to surround or bathe all tissues and increase blood volume when it joins the blood. A healthy lymphatic system works in harmony with the circulatory system to balance the fluids of the body. Excess fluid that is not absorbed by the blood capillaries is taken up by the lymphatic system where it is filtered and taken back to the heart.

There are about 500 to 1500 lymph nodes scattered throughout the human body. They are heavily concentrated in the neck, axilla (armpit), abdomen and groin. They range from the size of a pinhead to the size of a kidney bean. Lymph nodes contain lymphocytes (T and B cells), macrophage, plasma cells and accessory cells. Initial lymph vessels are found just under the skin. They trap fluids and large particles, especially proteins, from the interstitial tissue (the space between the tissue) into their finger-like projections. Once in the initial lymph vessels, the fluids and particles become lymph and cannot flow back to the interstitium. The lymph fluid becomes increasingly concentrated as it travels through the lymphatic system into larger, deeper collector vessels until it eventually reaches the lymph nodes. In the lymph nodes, bacteria, cell debris, and potential pathogens are filtered out of the lymph and destroyed by immune defense cells. After the lymph fluid is filtered, it drains into the lymphatic trunks and lymph ducts (thoracic duct or right lymphatic duct) and eventually into the heart to join the blood for circulation to the body.

The transport of the lymph fluid is affected by the movement of skeletal muscles, pulse of the arteries, breathing (pressure differences in the thorax), peristalsis (an involuntary wave-like contraction that propels the contents of the intestine forward) in the intestine, and the mechanoreceptors (receptors responding to touch or muscular movement) in the lymph vessel wall. This is why exercise, deep breathing and stretching are recommended for maintaining optimal lymphatic health. Lymphatic drainage massage is effective because it stimulates the mechanoreceptors in the lymph vessels.

Lymphatic drainage massage is used to manipulate the initial lymph vessels to facilitate transportation and direct the flow of interstitial fluid into the lymphatic system for circulation. Regional lymphatic trunks and nodes are massaged first in order to clear these pathways and to create a space for the lymph to flow into. The massage begins proximal (nearest to the centre or trunk of the body) and is extended outward in the direction of lymph flow. This means that with breast or chest surgery, the lymph nodes in the neck and axilla would be massaged first. If you undergo breast surgery for the treatment of cancer, a number of the axillary lymph nodes may also be removed. In this case, alternative pathways or watersheds (lines that divide lymph pathways or sections) are used to direct the flow of lymph into functional nodes such as the opposite axilla and abdominal nodes.

If you choose to include lymphatic drainage as part of your surgical support pre- or post-operatively, you will be required to complete a thorough health case history prior to treatment. Collaboration with the attending surgeon, patient and lymph drainage therapist is recommended to ensure that lymphatic drainage will be an effective treatment and does not pose any risk or potential harm to the patient.

Pre-Operative

Many people choose lymphatic drainage as part of their pre-operative care. As stated previously, lymphatic drainage facilitates the movement of lymph flow. This means that unwanted substances such as cell debris, potential pathogens and bacteria are moved from the interstitial tissue into the lymph nodes, where they are destroyed. It makes sense to try to eliminate as much "waste" as possible from our body before we have surgery. Generally, breast/chest lymphatic drainage would not be recommended for individuals with severe cardiac or kidney disease, acute infection (breast or systemic), or untreated cancer.

In some cases, after appropriate collaboration, a modified treatment may be implemented to meet your health needs and your particular surgery. For instance, if you are undergoing breast/chest surgery for the treatment of cancer, the breast or chest area with cancer could not be treated with lymphatic drainage but the other breast/chest could. Some therapists believe that treatment of the non-cancer side can reflexively affect the opposite side, although studies vary from supporting this perspective to indicating such treatment has no effect. These are generalizations only. Each person has to be thoroughly assessed prior to treatment. When to start treatment, how often to treat, duration, and so on is dependent upon your current health, your health history, and the type of and reason for surgery.

Post-Operative

Post-surgery lymphatic drainage can be quite helpful. Documented research has shown that babies (human and animal) need touch to thrive, and that injured tissue heals faster and more effectively when massaged. A series of specific, light massage strokes are performed on the neck, shoulder, and around the affected breast, chest and back to help reduce swelling and encourage lymph flow. A reduction in swelling or edema nearly always results in a reduction of pain. Utmost care is taken to avoid any pulling or direct contact with the surgical site until it is adequately healed and safe to do so. Lymphatic drainage can help promote optimal conditions for tissue regeneration by clearing away dead cells, debris and metabolites, thus enhancing the flow of oxygenated blood and nutrients.

Post-surgical infection can cause incredible pain and delay tissue healing. Part of the lymphatic drainage treatment is to observe patients for any signs of infection and to ensure that they do not develop cellulitis. Cellulitis is an inflammation of the skin and subcutaneous tissue due to an infection. Symptoms may include pain, redness and swelling. If your breast/chest incision is infected, lymphatic drainage on or close to the incision would not be recommended. Lymph drainage on or close to the infected area may spread an acute infection. You may also find touch on this area too painful or unwanted at the time. Lymph drainage treatments may resume when the infection is clear. Anyone who has or suspects they have cellulitis should seek medical attention. Antibiotics are effective in treating cellulitis.

"Lymphedema is defined as an abnormal accumulation of tissue proteins, edema, and chronic inflammation within an extremity."[1] It occurs when the lymphatic system does not work properly and can be either primary or secondary. Primary lymphedema is caused by a congenital disorder of the lymphatic system. Secondary lymphedema is caused by damage to the lymphatic system from injury, malignancy, scarring, infection or cancer treatments such as surgery, lymph node dissection and radiation. When lymphedema is a complication of breast cancer treatments, swelling usually occurs in the arm from which axillary lymph nodes were removed. As a result, the lymphatic system is compromised and cannot move excess fluid and particles out of the interstitial tissues fast enough to keep up with the production of lymph fluid. The result is swelling, impaired circulation and congestion. Lymphedema is a protein rich edema. This is significant because protein can be an excellent breeding ground for bacteria and infection. It is therefore extremely important for anyone who is at risk for lymphedema to be vigilant about watching for signs of infection on the at-risk arm. Some people who have lymphedema have found they have been able to manage their lymphedema through proper skin care, lymphatic drainage, and compression bandages or garments. Remember that not everyone who is at risk develops lymphedema. Many do not.

Anyone who is susceptible to lymphedema (lymph nodes removed or damaged, radiation therapy) should get as much information about it as possible. The following self-care is recommended:

1. Keep skin clean and dry. Clean even small wounds thoroughly. You may wish to carry a small tube of antibiotic cream and a couple of bandages with you.

2. Use gloves to protect your hands from cuts or burns when working or cooking.

3. Avoid invasive medical care on your at-risk or affected arm (needles, blood pressure cuffs, etc.).

4. Make note of any changes in your arm or chest. Be aware of feelings of heaviness, tingling, heat or tightness. Some people describe a feeling like an elastic band around the arm. These may be early signs of lymphedema. Consult your health-care practitioner.

5. Keep active. Exercise sensibly. Swimming, rebounding (mini-trampoline) and yoga can all help stimulate the lymphatic system.

In summary, manual lymph drainage is a gentle and non-invasive technique that may be beneficial in relation to breast or chest surgery pre-operatively, post-operatively, and in the management and treatment of lymphedema.

NOTE

1. M. Grabois, "Breast Cancer: Post-Mastectomy Lymphedema," *Physical Medical Rehabilitation* 8, no. 2 (1994), 267–77.

PAM HAMMOND is a registered massage therapist, shiatsu therapist and certified manual lymph drainage therapist and is currently in private practice in Toronto. She has worked as a clinical supervisor and teacher for over ten years. She is currently on the board of directors for Women's Healthy Environments Network.

Yoga and Breast Surgery

Esther Myers

The word yoga comes from the root "yuj" meaning "to yoke." It means integration, making whole by bringing all parts together, unifying. The practice is intended to enable us to experience the underlying coherence and interconnectedness within us, in our relationship to the world, and in the universe itself.

Yoga includes a myriad of techniques and practices, including ethical precepts, study, meditation, mantra and visualization, as well as the postures and breathing techniques which are best known in the West. They teach us to focus our attention within and attune to and be at ease in our bodies; to develop strength, flexibility, ease and grace of movement. These skills are useful when you are contemplating breast or chest surgery and in the recovery period.

If you are living in a large urban center, you have quite a wide selection of yoga classes and styles to choose from. They range from very strong, dynamic and physically demanding styles on the one hand, to slow, gentle, relaxing approaches on the other. This same variety and range is reflected in the many books and videotapes that are now on the market.

If you are looking for a yoga class, you may want to think about which of the various styles most suits your personality, rhythms and needs. The class should feel right for you.

- Do you want an active class to complement your current fitness program as a form of cross-training or are you looking for a slower, more relaxed and integrative environment?

- The more strenuous classes tend to attract younger and fitter students. What age group and level of fitness would most meet your needs?

- How much breathing practice or meditation would you like?

- Do you want a class with a strong spiritual focus like chanting or inspirational readings?

Yoga teachers vary hugely in background, training, experience and focus. Since you are considering breast or chest surgery, or may have already had an operation, you need to look for a teacher who understands the structure of the body well, and can adapt the poses to your needs, ability and energy. These will change over time as you recuperate.

Yoga practice doesn't take a lot of special equipment, or much space. You can do yoga just about anywhere. I have done it in hospital beds, in airports — all kinds of places. A quiet clear space that is relatively free of interruptions and distractions, of course, is ideal. You want to be comfortable and feel free to move so loose comfortable clothing is preferable. And you want to be really careful about how much you feel ready to do at any given time. It will depend on your energy, on how recently your surgery was, and whether you are receiving post-operative treatment.

The benefits of yoga practice, meditation relaxation and breathing practices increase with regularity. Even very short practices are beneficial if you do them regularly. Even five minutes of shoulder stretches, guided relaxation, or meditation helps. Every little bit makes a difference.

My teaching style is on the slow, integrative end of the spectrum. It begins with attention to the breath and a felt sense of stability on the ground.

Take a moment to become aware of your breathing, the rhythmic flow of your inhalation and exhalation. As you exhale, let go for a moment of any sense of busyness or effort.

Breath awareness is the foundation of many yoga and meditation practices. It is one of a number of underlying themes or principles that run through the entire practice. Our breath provides an immediate focus of attention that we can access easily because it is with us all the time. As you focus on your breathing you will notice how busy and active your mind is and where the tensions in your body are. Your emotions will all come to the surface. With time, this whirlwind subsides and we come into a quieter more reflective place. When I was diagnosed with breast cancer in 1994, I was grateful that my practice had taught me that it is possible to reach a quiet center, a place of inner knowing. I also knew that I should not make any decisions until I had reached that place. When I reached it, I would know what to do. I chose to have a mastectomy.

If, like me, you are facing cancer, then you have to make potentially irrevocable decisions in a very short time. At the same time, you are most likely riding an emotional roller coaster of shock, fear, anxiety, anger or terror. Especially at times like this, the capacity to stop and wait is invaluable. If you are considering elective chest or breast surgery, then you have much more time to reflect and to consider your options. There is a moment of exhalation, the "aha" moment when you are clear about the choice that is right for you.

Learning to be attuned to your body and your breathing is also extremely valuable after your operation. As soon as you wake up from the anaes-thetic, you can start to reconnect with your breath. Since movement in your upper body will be limited, focus on the rise and fall of your belly as you inhale and exhale. This abdominal breathing will help to reactivate your body. It is an on-going vehicle for tuning into your body and becoming reacquainted with the sensations and sensitivities. As you gradually regain movement and flexibility, the sensitivity that you develop through breath awareness will help you to know how much movement is appropriate at each stage of convalescence. Paying attention to your breathing is a powerful way of listening to your body. Let it tell you how much it is ready to move and to stretch, how strong it is, and what it is ready to do.

As your incision(s) heal, be aware of the movement of your chest as you breathe. The breath movement itself will gently stretch and revitalize the tissue. Scar tissue is generally tougher and less elastic than normal tissue. Residues of stiffness can remain for a long time after the surgery, so the process of freeing and normalizing the tissue is gradual and long-term.

Breast or chest surgery may well evoke psychological issues around your sexuality, either positive or negative. It may affect your relationships. The time you take quietly with your breath can help you come back to being at home with the changes in your body and self-image.

My teaching also focuses on developing a conscious sense of a secure physical foundation. When we feel more stable, we are more at ease and function better. This same logic applies to the body. When we can clearly feel a stable base on the ground, we relax. This awareness helps to rebuild confidence and improves posture as we recover from surgery and adapt to the changes in our body.

As you focus on your breathing, feel the support underneath you — the contact of your body with the chair, the couch, the bed, or the floor. Let yourself relax into that support. As you relax into the sensation of support, be aware of an underlying ground which, like the breath, is always there, when you take the time to notice.

When you are upright, sitting or standing, focus on your spine as a core support, like the trunk of a tree. Let this sense of verticality help you to emerge tall and free after your surgery.

Feel that your spine is supporting you. A sense of inner support or core support is something that we need all of the time, especially when we are healing.

I would like to conclude with a couple of simple shoulder movements that I have found helpful for myself and for others. Check with your doctor before you begin them.

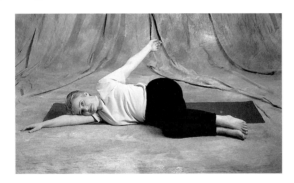

ARM CIRCLES: This exercise can be done in bed or on the floor. Lie on the side which is most comfortable. Curl up in a relaxed fetal position, with a pillow or folded blanket under your head.

Staying aware of your breathing, make circles with the free arm. Start slowly with small circles and gradually increase the circumference of the circles and the number of rotations. Practise both clockwise and counterclockwise.

Notice any tension or tenderness in and around the scar. As you breathe, let the movement gently stretch the tissue without straining or forcing. Let your body tell you how far it is ready to move.

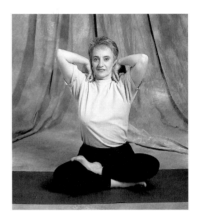

SITTING TWISTS: Sit comfortably with your spine as straight as possible. Put your hands on your shoulders so that your thumbs are pointing down your back and your fingers fan into your armpits.

Keeping your spine straight, slowly twist from side to side, exhaling as you go into the twist and inhaling as you come back to centre.

This movement stretches the front of the chest and the armpits, and releases the tension in the upper back between the shoulder blades. As before, go gently when you feel tension or tenderness.

With twenty-five years' teaching experience, ESTHER MYERS has a unique and organic approach to yoga and a deep understanding of its underlying rhythms and principles. Based in Toronto, Esther has given classes across Canada, in Europe and the United States, and has extensive experience training teachers. She is the author of Yoga & You *and produced a video on her teacher, Vanda Scaravelli. A breast-cancer survivor herself, her video,* Gentle Yoga for Breast Cancer Survivors, *was developed from her very successful yoga program at the Marvelle Koffler Breast Centre in Mt. Sinai Hospital.*

Surgical Information

Vladimir Lange and The American Society of Plastic Surgeons

The following chapter is based on information that has been provided by the American Society of Plastic Surgeons (Web site: www.plasticsurgery.org) and from chapters three and four of *Be A Survivor*™ — *Your Guide to Breast Cancer Treatment* (second edition) by Dr. Vladimir Lange.

If you are considering any of these surgeries, the information provided in this chapter will give you a basic understanding of the procedures. This information, however, can't answer all of your questions since a lot depends on your individual circumstances. Please ask your surgeon if there is anything you don't understand about the procedure you are considering. For more information on whether breast surgery is right for you, the initial consultation and what questions are important to ask, how to prepare for surgery, and what you can expect from your surgeon and surgery itself, refer to the American Society of Plastic Surgeons Web site above. For additional resources, refer to the Bibliography at the end of this book.

Breast Cancer Diagnosis and Staging

The only sure way to confirm a diagnosis of breast cancer is to perform a biopsy — that is, to remove a small piece of the tumour and have it examined under a microscope by a pathologist. The sample can be obtained either with a needle or surgically. If the tumour is small, or if there is a good possibility that it is not cancerous, your physician may choose either a fine needle aspiration or a core needle biopsy.

Fine Needle Aspiration

Fine needle aspiration, or FNA, is done with a very thin needle connected to a syringe. The needle is moved in and out several times to obtain the best sample possible. Even if no cancer cells are found, your doctor may want to have the lump removed surgically.

Core Needle Biopsy

Core needle biopsy is done with a larger needle, which can yield a larger sample. The procedure can be done under a local anaesthetic and takes only a few minutes. Most women who have had the procedure report only minor discomfort.

If the lesion is non-palpable (cannot be felt by hand), the core needle biopsy can be done using special mammography equipment (stereoctatic unit). This equipment enables the radiologist to place the needle precisely into the tumour, even if it is as small as a pea. The biopsy also can be done using ultrasound equipment. The choice generally depends on what your physician is most comfortable with.

The core biopsy itself is performed with a device that works like an ear-piercing instrument: it propels a needle very rapidly through the lesion. A special notch in the needle traps a sliver of tissue for examination. Samples obtained with core biopsy are large enough to be cut into thin slices and examined under the microscope, providing a diagnosis that some doctors feel is more reliable than that from an FNA.

A new device is the Mammotome system that uses a small rotating cutter and vacuum to move an even larger sample. This leads to a reliable diagnosis and the need for fewer insertions of the needle.

Surgical Biopsy

Another way your doctor may choose to obtain a biopsy is surgically. A surgical biopsy is performed under local or general anaesthesia. Most surgical biopsies are excisional, in which the surgeon removes the entire tumour.

The surgical biopsy takes about an hour, and causes minimal post-operative pain that goes away in a few days. You can usually begin doing non-strenuous work the day after the biopsy, although you should not lift heavy objects for a few weeks. The incision usually heals within ten days.

Lumpectomy or Partial Mastectomy

If the tumour is small and confined to a single location in the breast, you may have the option of having breast-conserving surgery. The goal of this relatively simple procedure is to remove the whole tumour, while conserving as much breast tissue as possible. A margin of normal breast tissue of about one-half to three quarters of an inch in thickness is also removed to make sure no malignant cells are left behind. Depending on how much breast tissue is removed, the procedure may also be called wide excision, segmental mastectomy, or quadrantectomy. The specific technique used may vary from surgeon to surgeon and from case to case. The cosmetic result of breast-conserving surgery will vary with the location and size of the tumour, and the size of the breast. A few very large tumours may be treated first with chemotherapy or radiation in order to shrink them before being removed surgically. Breast-conserving surgery almost always requires additional treatment of the breast area

with high energy x-rays (radiation therapy) to reduce the chance that any surviving cancer cells are left behind.

A lumpectomy takes about an hour. The surgeon will make a skin incision over the tumour area and remove the tumour with a small amount of surrounding healthy breast tissue. The surgical specimen will be sent to a pathologist who will examine it under a microscope and determine whether the margins are clear of tumour cells. If tumour cells are found along the edges (dirty margins), it means that some cancerous cells may have been left behind. Another lumpectomy may be done to get clear margins. In some cases, a mastectomy may be required.

Mastectomy

Mastectomy, or surgical removal of the breast, has been used to treat breast cancer for over a century. The radical mastectomy — which removed the entire breast, the lymph nodes in the armpit, and one of the major muscles of the chest wall — was based on the assumption that the more tissue removed, the better the chances of curing the cancer.

In the 1970s and 1980s, research proved that there was no advantage in removing the chest muscles, and the modified radical mastectomy, which spares these muscles, yielding a more cosmetically acceptable result, was introduced. Now the radical mastectomy is almost never performed. Today's modified radical mastectomy removes as much of the breast tissue as possible, including the nipple and areola, and a number of axillary lymph nodes, but not the muscles. Patients can choose from a variety of reconstruction techniques.

The total mastectomy takes two to three hours. Breast tissue extends from the collar bone to the edge of the ribs, and from the breast bone to the muscles in the back of the armpit. The surgeon will make an elliptical incision to separate the breast from the chest wall, then remove as much of the breast tissue as possible. The tissue will be sent to the pathologist, who will examine it for any evidence of cancer spread beyond the breast.

Unless your tumour was very small, you also may have an axillary lymph node dissection — removal of a number of lymph nodes from your armpit for examination by the pathologist. Presence or absence of cancer cells in these lymph nodes will help determine your future treatments.

If you've decided to have immediate reconstruction of the breast, the plastic surgeon will take over while you are still asleep. Reconstruction can be done using your own tissues — from the abdomen, back, or buttocks, or using a synthetic implant. The procedure may take anywhere from an hour to six or eight hours, depending on the method used.

When the procedure (mastectomy or node dissection) is completed, one or two tubes called "drains" will be placed under the skin to help drain the fluid that accumulates at the site of surgery. If you go home with the drains, you'll receive instructions on how to care for them.

Breast Reconstruction Following Breast Removal

Almost every woman who has lost a breast to cancer is eligible for breast reconstruction, however the following conditions are desirable: You clearly understand that your reconstructed breast will not look or feel exactly the same as the breast that was removed. Your oncologist has advised you that reconstruction is appropriate for you with regard to your stage of cancer or treatment. You feel that you are able to handle the period of emotional adjustment that may accompany breast reconstruction. Just as it takes time to get used to the loss of a breast, it may take some time before you begin to think of the reconstructed breast as your own. You have no additional health concerns that may complicate the procedure, such as obesity or heart disease.

There are many options available in breast reconstruction. Your anatomy, your surgeon's preferences and your desired results will help determine which method is best for you.

Skin Expansion with a Breast Implant

This is the most common method of reconstructing a breast. Following mastectomy, a balloon expander is inserted beneath the skin and chest muscle. Over several weeks, the expander balloon is gradually filled with a salt-water solution in the doctor's office, causing the overlying skin to stretch. When the skin has stretched sufficiently, the expander is surgically replaced with a more permanent implant. Some expanders are designed to be left in place as the final implant. The nipple and the areola are reconstructed in a later procedure. In rare cases, when a sufficient amount of skin is available, an implant can be placed without the preliminary skin-expansion step.

Flap Reconstruction

Although flap reconstruction is more involved at the initial procedure than reconstruction with an implant, many women prefer it because it may allow the breast to be rebuilt with natural tissue. Also, unlike the tissue-expander method, the breast mound is completed at the initial operation, without the need for expansion over an extended time period.

In one method, the breast is reconstructed using a tissue flap — consisting of a portion of skin, fat and muscle — that is taken from the back or abdomen. The flap, still tethered to its original blood supply, is tunneled beneath the skin to the front of the chest wall. The transported tissue may be bulky enough to create a new breast mound itself. However, sometimes an implant will be inserted as well.

In a more complex flap technique, tissue that is removed from the abdomen, is surgically transplanted to the chest by reconnecting the flap's blood vessels to vessels in the chest region. Although more complicated, this micro-surgical reconstruction may provide a more natural and less traumatic reconstruction in many women.

Although recovery from flap reconstruction may take longer than with implant reconstruction at the initial procedure, it does not require a secondary procedure for placing a permanent implant, nor does it require the weekly office visits needed for tissue expansion.

All of these procedures have advantages and disadvantages, and many times the choice of procedures is limited by other health factors, such as weight, other medical conditions and previous cancer therapy. Your plastic surgeon will help you to determine which is the best procedure for you.

Follow-up Procedures

Once the breast mound is restored in the initial procedure, one or more follow-up procedures will be performed to replace the tissue expander with a permanent implant or to reconstruct the nipple and areola. Your surgeon may also recommend an additional operation to lift or reduce the opposite breast to match the appearance of the reconstructed breast.

Risks

Certain complications, including blood loss, infection and others, are possible in any type of surgery. Potential complications specific to breast reconstruction vary with the type of reconstruction you and your surgeon choose. For instance, with flap reconstruction, there is a small risk of partial or, very rarely, complete flap loss. Reconstruction with an implant has the potential for breast firmness (capsular contracture) and implant rupture. The probability of having one of these or other complications as well as your specific risk must be thoroughly discussed with your surgeon.

Breast Reduction

Breast reduction, or reduction mammoplasty, is a procedure that removes excess breast tissue and skin. The areola may be reduced and repositioned as well. Having the procedure will give you more than just smaller, firmer breasts. Patients also experience significant relief from many physical and emotional discomforts, and a new sense of freedom in exercise and physical activity. Of all the procedures that plastic surgeons perform, breast reduction ranks among the highest in patient satisfaction.

Breast reduction can be performed at any age, but plastic surgeons usually recommend waiting until breast development has stopped. Childbirth and breast-feeding may affect the size and shape of your breasts. If you plan to breast-feed in the future, you should discuss this with your surgeon.

The Surgery

The specific method chosen for your breast reduction will be determined by your anatomy, your surgeon's preferences and your desired results. The most common method uses a three-part incision. One part of the incision is made around the areola. Another runs vertically from the bottom edge of the areola to the crease underneath the breast. The third part is a horizontal incision beneath the breast, which follows the natural curve of the breast crease. After the surgeon has removed the excess breast tissue, fat and skin, the nipple and areola are reduced in size. Skin that was formerly located above the nipple is brought down and together to reshape the breast. Liposuction may be used to improve the contour, especially on the sides of the breasts. The nipples and areolae usually remain attached to their underlying tissue as they are moved to their higher position and this may allow for the preservation of sensation. This method may also preserve the ability to breast-feed, although it is not guaranteed. The type of incision used for your breast reduction may vary, depending on the size and shape of your breasts and the desired amount of reduction. Women who seek a smaller reduction in size may be able to avoid the horizontal incision that runs underneath the breast. Other incisional techniques may be used in some instances. Women whose breasts contain a significant amount of fatty tissue may find that liposuction alone can be used to reduce breast size with only minimal scars.

Breast Reduction for Men and Liposuction

Gynaecomastia is a medical term that comes from the Greek words for "woman-like breasts." Though this oddly named condition is rarely talked about, it's actually quite common. Gynaecomastia affects an estimated 40 to 60 percent of men. It may affect only one breast or both. Though certain drugs and medical problems have been linked with male breast overdevelopment, there is no known cause in the vast majority of cases. The procedure removes fat and/or glandular tissues from the breasts, and in extreme cases removes excess skin.

The best candidates for surgery have firm, elastic skin that will reshape to the body's new contours. Surgery may be discouraged for obese men, or for overweight men who have not first attempted to correct the problem with exercise or weight loss. Also, individuals who drink alcohol beverages in excess or smoke marijuana are usually not considered good candidates for surgery. These drugs, along with anabolic steroids, may cause gynaecomastia. Therefore, patients

are first directed to stop the use of these drugs to see if the breast fullness will diminish before surgery is considered an option.

Risks

When male breast reduction surgery is performed by a qualified plastic surgeon, complications are infrequent and usually minor. Nevertheless, as with any surgery, there are risks. These include infection, skin injury, excessive bleeding, adverse reaction to anaesthesia, and excessive fluid loss or accumulation. The procedure may also result in noticeable scars, permanent pigment changes in the breast area, or slightly mismatched breasts or nipples. If asymmetry is significant, a second procedure may be performed to remove additional tissue. The temporary effects of breast reduction include loss of breast sensation or numbness, which may last up to a year.

The Surgery

If excess glandular tissue is the primary cause of the breast enlargement, it will be excised, or cut out, with a scalpel. The excision may be performed alone or in conjunction with liposuction. In a typical procedure, an incision is made in an inconspicuous location — either on the edge of the areola or in the under arm area. Working through the incision, the surgeon cuts away the excess glandular tissue, fat and skin from around the areola and from the sides and bottom of the breast. Major reductions that involve the removal of a significant amount of tissue and skin may require larger incisions that result in more conspicuous scars. If the liposuction is used to remove excess fat, the cannula is usually inserted through the existing incisions.

If your gynaecomastia consists primarily of excessive fatty tissue, your surgeon will likely use liposuction to remove the excess fat. A small incision, less than half-inch in length, is made around the edge of the areola, or the incision may be placed in the underarm area. A slim hollow tube called a cannula, which is attached to the vacuum pump, is then inserted into the incision. Using strong, deliberate strokes, the surgeon moves the cannula through the layers beneath the skin, breaking up the fat and suctioning it out. Patients may feel a vibration or some friction during the procedure, but generally no pain. In extreme cases where large amounts of fat or glandular tissue have been removed, skin may not adjust well to the new smaller breast contour, requiring the removal of some skin to allow it to readjust to the new breast contour.

Sometimes, a small drain is inserted through a separate incision to draw off excess fluids. Once closed, the incisions are usually covered with a dressing. The chest may be wrapped to keep the skin firmly in place.

Breast Augmentation

Breast augmentation, technically know as augmentation mammoplasty, is a surgical procedure to enhance the size and shape of a woman's breasts. By inserting an implant behind each breast, the surgery can increase a woman's bust-line by one or more bra cup sizes.

Types of Implants

A breast implant is a silicone shell filled with either silicone gel or a salt-water solution known as saline. Because of concerns that there is insufficient information demonstrating the safety of silicone gel-filled breast implants, the American Food & Drug Administration (FDA) has determined that new gel-filled implants, at the present time, should be available only to women participating in approved studies. Some women requiring replacement of the implants may also be eligible to participate in the study. Saline-filled implants continue to be available to breast augmentation patients in the United States on an unre-

stricted basis, pending further FDA review. You should ask your doctor more about the specifics of the FDA decisions. For the most recent research on types of implants, check the Canadian and American Web sites mentioned in the Bibliography.

Risks

The most common problem, capsular contracture, occurs if the scar or capsule around the implant begins to tighten. This squeezing of the soft implant can cause the breast to feel hard. Capsular contracture can be treated in several ways, and sometimes requires either removal or "scoring" of the scar tissue, or perhaps removal or replacement of the implant.

Excessive bleeding following the operation may cause some swelling and pain. If excessive bleeding continues, another operation may be needed to control the bleeding and remove the accumulated blood.

A small percentage of women develop an infection around an implant. This may occur at any time, but is most often seen within a week after surgery. In some cases, the implant may need to be removed for several months until the infection clears. A new implant can then be inserted.

Some women report that their nipples become over-sensitive, under-sensitive, or even numb. You may also notice small patches of numbness near your incisions. These symptoms usually disappear within time, but may be permanent in some patients.

There is no evidence that breast implants will affect fertility, pregnancy, or your ability to nurse. If, however, you have nursed a baby within the year before augmentation, you may produce milk for a few days after surgery. This may cause some discomfort, but can be treated with medication prescribed by your doctor.

Breast implants may break or leak. Rupture can occur as a result of injury or even from the normal compression and movement of your breast and implant, causing the man-made shell to leak. If a saline-filled implant breaks, the implant will deflate in a few hours and the salt water will be harmlessly absorbed by the body.

If a break occurs in a gel-filled implant, however, one of two things may occur. If the shell breaks but the scar also breaks or tears, especially following extreme pressure, silicone gel may move into surrounding tissue. The gel may collect in the breast and cause a new scar to form around it, or it may migrate to another area of the body. There may be a change in the shape or firmness of the breast. Both types of breaks may require a second operation and replacement of the leaking implant. In some cases, it may not be possible to remove all of the silicone gel in the breast tissue if a rupture should occur.

A few women with breast implants have reported symptoms similar to diseases of the immune system, such as scleroderma and other arthritis-like conditions. These symptoms may include joint pain or swelling, fever, fatigue, or breast pain. Research has found no clear link between silicone breast implants and the symptoms of what doctors refer to as "connective-tissue disorders," but the FDA in the United States has requested further study.

While there is no evidence that breast implants cause breast cancer, they may change the way mammography is done to detect cancer. When you request a routine mammogram, be sure to go to a radiology center where technicians are experienced in the special techniques required to get a reliable x-ray of a breast with an implant. Additional views will be required. Ultrasound examinations may be of benefit in some women with implants to detect breast lumps or to evaluate the implant.

You should discuss each of these complications with your physician to make sure you understand the risks and consequences of breast augmentation.

Additional information for research is available in the Bibliography.

The Surgery

The method of inserting and positioning your implant will depend on your anatomy and your surgeon's recommendation. The incision can be made either in the crease where the breast meets the chest, around the areola (the dark skin surrounding the nipple), or in the armpit. Working through the incision, the surgeon will lift your breast tissue and skin to create a pocket, either directly behind the breast tissue or underneath your chest wall muscle (the pectoral muscle). The implants are then centered beneath your nipples.

Some surgeons believe that putting the implants behind your chest muscle may reduce the potential for capsular contracture. Drainage tubes may be used for several days following the surgery. This placement may also interfere less with breast examination by mammogram than if the implant is placed directly behind the breast tissue. Placement behind the muscle however, may be more painful for a few days after surgery than placement directly under the breast tissue.

You'll want to discuss the pros and cons of these alternatives with your doctor before surgery to make sure you fully understand the implications of the procedure he or she recommends for you.

The surgery usually takes one to two hours to complete. Stitches are used to close the incisions, which may also be taped for greater support. A gauze bandage may be applied over your breasts to help with healing.

Physician/producer/author VLADIMIR LANGE, *MD. combines his
medical education, clinical experience and communication talents
as the head of a leading company in the field of breast health.
Dr. Lange, a graduate of Harvard Medical School, practised
emergency medicine for thirteen years. He founded Lange
Productions in 1985 in order to combine his love of audiovisual
and print communications with his medical background to educate millions of patients and physicians world-wide. The
company's videos, CD-ROMs and books have been translated
into a dozen languages, and have been honored with many
awards for artistic excellence.*

Dr. Lange's book, Be A Survivor™ — Your Guide to Breast
Cancer Treatment *(second edition), is the outgrowth of his wife's
personal experience with breast cancer which highlighted the need
for clear, concise, yet comprehensive medical information for
patients and their families.*

BIBLIOGRAPHY

This bibliography is provided as a springboard to assist you in your research concerning breast or chest surgery. Print, video and Internet resources are listed below on a range of topics relevant to breast and chest surgery. You may also want to review the endnotes in the Journey to Healing: Health Care chapters as a further source of reference material. The resources listed here range from community support organizations to medical information to on-line chat resources. We have attempted to provide information from a variety of perspectives as well as on a range of topics.

PRINT RESOURCES

Anderson, Kim. *A Recognition of Being: Reconstructing Native Womanhood.* Toronto: Sumach Press, 2001.

Auckweiler, Becky, RN, MS. *Living in the Postmastectomy Body: Learning to Live In and Love Your Body Again.* Point Roberts, WA: Hartley & Marks, 1998.

Bertucci, Patricia. *Cancer Rage: A Photographic Journal of My Breast Cancer Experience.* Funded by Canadian Breast Cancer Foundation. Toronto: self-published, Patricia Bertucci Publisher, 2001.

Bondurant, Stuart, Ernster Virginia L., Herdman, Roger, editors. *Safety of Silicone Breast Implants.* Washington, DC: Institute of Medicine, National Academy Press, 2000.

Boyle, Wade and Saine, Andre. *Lectures in Naturopathic Hydrotherapy.* Sandy, Oregon: Eclectic Medical Publications, 1988.

Brownworth, Victoria A. *Coming Out of Cancer: Writings from the Lesbian Cancer Epidemic,* Seattle: Seal Press, 2000.

Burt, Jeannie, and White, Gwen, P.T. *Lymphedema: A Breast Cancer Patient's Guide to Prevention and Healing.* Alameda, CA: Hunter House Publishers, 1999.

Chart, Pamela, MD. *Breast Cancer: A Guide for Patients.* Toronto: Prospero Books, 2000.

Curties, Debra, RMT. *Breast Massage.* New Brunswick: Curties-Overzet Publications, 1999.

Kaur, Sat Dharam. *A Call To Women: The Healthy Breast Program and Workbook.* Kingston: Quarry Press Inc., 2000.

Labriola, Dan, ND. *Complementary Cancer Therapies: Combining Traditional and Alternative Approaches for the Best Possible Outcome.* Roseville, CA: Prima Health, 1999.

Lange, Vladimir, MD. *Be A Survivor™ — Your Guide to Breast Cancer Treatment.* Second edition. Los Angeles: Lange Productions, 1998.

Love, Susan, MD and Lindsay, Karen. *Dr. Susan Love's Breast Book.* Third edition. Reading: Perseus, 2002.

Olivotto, Ivor, MD, Gelmon, Karen, MD and Kuusk, Urve, MD. *Intelligent Patient Guide to Breast Cancer: All You Need to Know to Take an Active Part in Your Treatment.* Third Edition. Vancouver: Intelligent Patient Guide, 2001.

Redden, John. "Introduction to the Ancient Art of Poulticing," *Canadian Journal of Herbalism,* vol. xxiii no. 2, 2002: 8–12.

Weed, Susun S. *Breast Cancer? Breast Health!* Woodstock, New York: Ash Tree Publishing, 1996.

Weed, Susun S. *Healing Wise.* Woodstock, New York: Ash Tree Publishing, 1989.

West, Diana. *Defining Your Own Success: Breastfeeding after Breast Reduction Surgery.* Schaumburg, IL: La Leche League, 2001.

Williams, Penelope. *Alternatives in Cancer Therapy: The Case for Choice.* Toronto: Key Porter, 2000.

VIDEO

Myers, Esther. *Gentle Yoga for Breast Cancer Survivors.* Esther Myers, Explorations In Yoga, Inc., 2000. Order through www.estheryoga.com

INTERNET AND COMMUNITY RESOURCES

American Boyz, Inc (transmen): www.amboyz.org

American Society of Plastic Surgeons: www.plasticsurgery.org

ASTT(é)Q-Action Santé: Travesti(e)s et Transsexuel(le)s du Quebec: email assteq@sympatico.ca; phone (514)847-0067

Breast Cancer Action Nova Scotia: www.bca.ns.ca

Breast Cancer Action Saskatchewan: www.bcas.ca

Breast Health Access for Women with Disabilities: www.bhawd.org

Breastfeeding After Reduction (La Leche League site): www.bfar.org

Canadian Breast Cancer Foundation: www.cbcf.org

Canadian Breast Cancer Network: www.cbcn.ca

Canadian Breast Cancer Research Initiative: www.breast.cancer.ca

Cancer Information Services (Canadian Cancer Society): www.cancer.ca

Dr. Anne Lawrence – Transsexual Women's Resources: www.annelawrence.com

Feminist Women's Health Centre (USA): www.fwhc.org

Feminist.com (women's health & sexuality information) (USA): www.feminist.com/resources

Fondation Quebecois du cancer: www.fqc.qc.ca

Gynecomastia.org (USA): www.gynecomastia.org

John W Nick Foundation on Male Breast Cancer (USA): www.johnwnickfoundation.org

Male Breast Cancer Information, Marvelle Koffler Breast Centre (Mt. Sinai Hospital): www.mtsinai.on.ca/mkbc/mkbcresources/malebc.htm

Mindfully.org (nonprofit research site) (USA): www.mindfully.org/Health/Breast-Implant-Risks-FDA.html

National Breast Cancer Coalition (USA): www.natlbcc.org

National Cancer Institute/NCI (USA): www.nci.nih.gov

National Center for Policy Research for Women and Families (USA): www.center4policy.org

Ontario Breast Cancer Community Research Initiative (Toronto Sunnybrook Regional Cancer Centre): angela.sardelis@tsrcc.on.ca

Silicone Gel Breast Implants(UK): www.silicone-review.gov.uk

Silicone Survivors (USA): www.siliconesurvivors.net

Supportive Care (post breast surgery therapy rehabilitation exercises): www.cancersupportivecare.com/breastexercise.html

SusanLoveMD.com — The Website for Women (USA): www.SusanLoveMD.com

The 519 Church St. Community Centre: Meal Trans Program and Trans · Youth · Toronto! www.icomm.ca/the519/programs

The International Journal of Transgenderism: www.symposion.com/ijt

The TransBoy Resource Network: www.geocities.com/WestHollywood/Park/6484/

US Food & Drug Administration — Center for Devices & Radiological Health (breast implant information): www.fda.gov/cdrh/breastimplants

Wellspring Cancer Support (Ontario): www.wellspring.ca

Willow Breast Cancer Support & Resource Services: www.willow.org